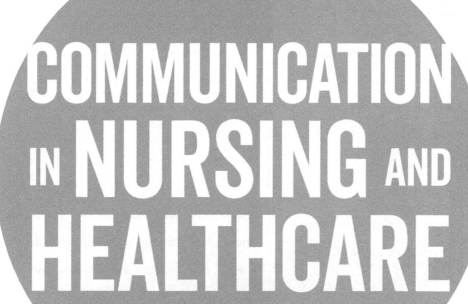

COMMUNICATION IN NURSING AND HEALTHCARE

A Guide for Compassionate Practice

IRIS GAULT, JEAN SHAPCOTT, ARMIN LUTHI AND GRAEME REID

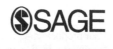

SAGE

Los Angeles | London | New Delhi
Singapore | Washington DC | Melbourne

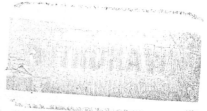

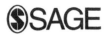

SAGE

Los Angeles | London | New Delhi
Singapore | Washington DC | Melbourne

SAGE Publications Ltd
1 Oliver's Yard
55 City Road
London EC1Y 1SP

SAGE Publications Inc.
2455 Teller Road
Thousand Oaks, California 91320

SAGE Publications India Pvt Ltd
B 1/I 1 Mohan Cooperative Industrial Area
Mathura Road
New Delhi 110 044

SAGE Publications Asia-Pacific Pte Ltd
3 Church Street
#10-04 Samsung Hub
Singapore 049483

Editor: Becky Taylor
Editorial assistant: Charlène Burin
Production editor: Katie Forsythe
Copyeditor: Sharon Cawood
Proofreader: Audrey Scriven
Indexer: Gary Kirby
Marketing manager: Camille Richmond
Cover design: Wendy Scott
Typeset by: C&M Digitals (P) Ltd, Chennai, India
Printed and bound by CPI Group (UK) Ltd,
Croydon, CR0 4YY

Library of Congress Control Number: 2016935331

British Library Cataloguing in Publication data

A catalogue record for this book is available from
the British Library

ISBN 978-1-4739-2669-1
ISBN 978-1-4129-6231-5 (pbk)

At SAGE we take sustainability seriously. Most of our products are printed in the UK using FSC papers and boards.
When we print overseas we ensure sustainable papers are used as measured by the PREPS grading system.
We undertake an annual audit to monitor our sustainability.

Table of Contents

Activities on the Values Exchange community website for this book –
http://sagecomms.vxcommunity.com

Student story 1.2: Jack
Critical thinking exercise 1.2: Communication – the basics
Critical thinking exercise 2.4: Social media and the internet
Critical debate 2.1: Reflection on communication – a TV interaction
Student story 3.1: Gemma
Critical thinking exercise 4.3. Motivational interviewing questions and thinking
    about behaviour change
Patient story 5.2: Lack of empathy
Student story 6.1: John
Patient story 6.1: The secret schizophrenic
Student (and patient) story 6.3: 'Life-changing care'
Critical thinking exercise 7.1. Reduced capacity to communicate
Nursing story 7.1: (Mis)interpretations of behaviour
Critical thinking exercise 8.2 Gillick competence
Critical thinking exercise 8.3 Thinking about young people
Student story 9.1: Difficulty in relating to older people
Critical thinking exercise 9.4: Mid Staffs public inquiry
Critical thinking exercise 10.1 Dealing with anger
Student story 11.1: Return to Gemma
Critical thinking exercise 11.4. Scenario – the 'troublesome' HCA
Student story 12.1: Return to Josh
Student story 12.2: Return to Molly
Critical thinking exercise 12.5: Moral disengagement

About the Authors

Iris Gault is a registered general and mental health nurse and worked in both settings following qualification. She has extensive experience in community mental healthcare and in nursing education. At the present time she is Associate Professor of mental health nursing in the Faculty of Health, Social Care and Education at Kingston University and St George's University of London. Her main interests lie in service user involvement and shared decision making around medication issues in mental health. She has published in this area and current projects include studies into Black, Asian and minority ethnic group perspectives on medication and on attitudes and knowledge regarding physical health skill development of mental health nurses.

Jean Shapcott is a registered children's nurse. She is a Senior Lecturer in children's nursing the Faculty of Health, Social Care and Education at Kingston University and St George's University of London. She has extensive experience in children's healthcare and in nursing education. She has published in the areas of communication and nurse education. Her research interests are in interprofessional practice and education; care of children with complex conditions; children's palliative care; technology enhanced learning.

Armin Luthi is a registered mental health nurse. He is a Senior Lecturer in mental health and mental health nursing at the Faculty of Health Care Sciences at London South Bank University. He has extensive experience in forensic mental health services and the delivery of cognitive therapies, both in practice and in education. He is currently developing a longitudinal study into the development of supported learning to facilitate emotional resilience in student nurses as well as researching the impact of mindfulness on the new nursing curriculum

Graeme Reid is a registered mental health nurse and was a mental health nursing student at the Faculty of Health, Social Care and Education at Kingston University and St George's University of London when the writing of this book commenced. Whilst other students contributed, Graeme provided the major component of the student nurse perspective on what is needed in communication skills for healthcare students. He has worked as a staff nurse in acute mental health nursing and is now working as a community psychiatric nurse within an early intervention in psychosis team.

Judith Francois is a registered general nurse and health visitor. She is a Senior Lecturer in the Clinical Leadership and Management team in nursing at the Faculty of Health, Social Care and Education at Kingston University and St George's University of London. She has extensive experience in community healthcare, in nursing education and has worked extensively with a range of families and individuals within the community setting, focusing on improving health. She has also worked with the NHS Leadership Academy on the Mary Seacole programme, and has a special interest in leadership, coaching and widening participation.

Introduction

Contemporary healthcare is radically changing in form, structure and expectation. The challenge is to improve health in people with multiple morbidities within a better integrated care environment and to manage a variety of complex situations. The health practitioner is required to communicate to promote health, to enable self-management with service users, to provide support in crisis and to effectively function in multi-agency and disciplinary environments. Contemporary healthcare requires an in-depth understanding of the influences on human behaviour and communicative methods that enable positive change to occur.

This book has been written with the aid of substantial input and advice from students. One of the authors, now qualified, began the process of writing the book whilst still a student nurse. Prior to the commissioning of the book, we asked healthcare students for their thoughts and opinions on what was needed in a book on communication. A focus group of third-year students at Kingston University and St George's University of London provided some 'very real' perspectives on what they felt was needed in a book on communication. However, in particular, students said that it was the 'difficult communication or conversations' in healthcare that really required addressing. Students in the latter stages of their training report difficulty in dealing with complex communication in their practice. Their feedback suggested that communication skills education was often focused on the earlier stages of courses. Nevertheless, they felt that they required more input for those occasions when facing patients with life-threatening/changing conditions, acute psychological distress or in need of assistance in changing problematic health behaviour. Therefore, we hope we have faithfully reflected these issues within the book.

This book is a text on communication, designed for student nurses and midwives to use throughout their three-year training in any field of healthcare practice. It aims to enable students to develop key, evidence-based therapeutic communication skills for today's healthcare settings. The book aims to help students understand the essential elements of compassionate communication, the theoretical underpinning, the techniques and tools to equip them to be competent practitioners. It will encourage students to be thoughtful, mindful and inquiring; capable of compassionate communication and collaborative partnerships with patients. The intention is to guide students from basic communication skills through to a more sophisticated understanding of how to enhance positive behaviour change, to cope with acute distress and negotiate within and across boundaries.

However, crucially the book also emphasises the importance of and provides tools to allow students to look after their own emotional wellbeing. Our view is that the majority of healthcare students commence their education with the intention of being compassionate and collaborative. Where compassion is found to be lacking, it is often the case that those practitioners have become overwhelmed and unable to attend to their own and their patients' emotional needs. Therefore, the book focuses as much on the student as it does on the patient or care group.

Structurally, the book is in three parts, developing in complexity and reflecting the stages of nurse and midwifery education. Part 1 concentrates on values and self-awareness; Part 2 on communication with specific care groups; and Part 3 on issues of importance as students face qualification. The terms 'patient' and 'service user' will be used interchangeably, reflecting the current reality of vocabulary within caring services.

PART 1

FUNDAMENTALS OF COMMUNICATION FOR COMPASSIONATE PRACTICE

Part 1 is designed to help students develop a better understanding of themselves within the context of healthcare. It aims to allow them to explore their communicative and collaborative abilities in order to more effectively apply these to their patients. Whilst there is some discussion of 'how to do communication', the emphasis is on examining the factors influencing underlying attitudes towards ourselves and others. This section will refer to patients and clinical scenarios but the focus is on the individual practitioner. It illustrates how theory and contemporary psychological applications can enhance coping mechanisms, communication and collaborative skills for student nurses and midwives.

Chapter 1 looks at understanding the context of communicative and compassionate care. It examines the centrality of communication to collaborative relationships and the values underpinning care. Chapter 2 explores the components of professional communication in nursing and midwifery and begins to introduce the student to an understanding of reflective practice. Chapter 3 looks at the developmental psychological theory of Piaget and Bowlby. These important psychological building blocks help develop an appreciation of the processes that affect our own and others' behaviour and communication patterns. Chapter 4 highlights contemporary health issues and the need to develop more effective forms of health behaviour change methods. Part 1 then concludes with emotional intelligence/competence and mindfulness; acknowledging that it is essential that nurses and midwives look after their own psychological wellbeing, in order to effectively communicate and collaboratively care for patients and service users.

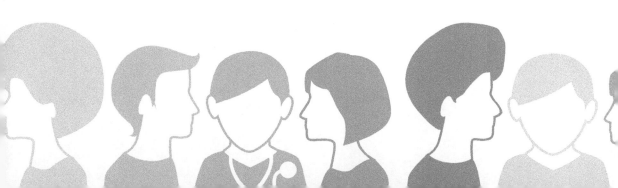

1

Essential Values for Communication, Compassion and Collaborative Care

Iris Gault, Graeme Reid and Armin Luthi

• • • • • • • • • • • • Learning Objectives • • • • • • • • • • • •

By the end of this chapter, you will have developed an understanding of:

- the importance of communication and the context of failures in compassionate communication and care
- the ethical values underpinning compassionate communication: respect and preservation of dignity
- the complexity and centrality of the therapeutic relationship.

Don't forget to visit the Values Exchange website at http://sagecomms.vxcommunity.com for extra practice and revision activities.

• •

Introduction

Nationally and internationally the requirement for nurses to communicate effectively and ethically is highlighted and documented in essential standards and codes of behaviour. In the United Kingdom, the Nursing and Midwifery Council's standards for pre-registration nursing state:

> All nurses must build partnerships and therapeutic relationships through safe, effective and non-discriminatory communication. They must take account of individual differences, capabilities and needs

and

They must ensure people receive all the information they need in a language and manner that allows them to make informed choices and share decision making. (Nursing and Midwifery Council England, 2010, p. 15)

In this chapter, we argue that in order to achieve the standards expected in the effective delivery of healthcare, it is crucial to fully understand the importance of compassion, apparent failures in compassion, the ethical values underpinning positive communication and the centrality and complexity of communication in therapeutic relationships. It is also necessary to appreciate that a seemingly simple task such as communicating with a patient is actually a complex and skilled process. This chapter unpicks the intricacies of communication and encourages the student to maintain an inquiring approach to practice that might look undemanding at first glance.

The importance of communication and remaining compassionate

Will you remain compassionate and caring in your communication?

Student story 1.1: Janet

Janet is a first-year student nurse. She is one of the more mature students at 35 but is full of enthusiasm for her career change and considers herself to be a 'people person'. She used to work in a high-powered job in finance and, had she stayed, would certainly have earned more money than she ever will in nursing. However, she became disillusioned with finance, feeling that a lifestyle associated with simply earning money was not for her. Consequently, she has given up a lot to be a student nurse and hopes it will all work out. She is married and has two children who are now half way through secondary school, so this seems a good time to make the change. Her husband and children are supportive of her doing a nursing course. She feels a bit anxious about learning the technical aspects of the job but thinks she is making progress. Janet has just started her first placement on a busy medical ward. She's enjoying the work but notices that because she looks older than the other first years (they are both 19), the patients seem to expect her to be able to provide reassurance in a way that they don't expect from the younger students. In addition, when the practice educator comes round and sees all of the students in a group, the younger students always seem to expect her to answer first when they are asked a question. It's all a bit more difficult than she expected.

　　She's also very aware that just as she has entered nursing, there is a lot of publicity about poor standards of care. Janet is very determined that she will maintain her own high standards but she recognises that the ward is very busy (it is winter and lots of older people are being admitted) and she can also see that some of the healthcare assistants are cutting corners.

Student story 1.2: Jack

Jack is a first-year learning disability student nurse. He had worked as a support worker in learning disabilities prior to commencing his nursing course. Jack is 33; he took quite a while to work out what he wanted to do in life. He started a sociology degree in his 20s but felt it wasn't for him and did not complete the course. He has had a number of jobs in sales but, again, felt that it wasn't for him. A friend worked as a residential social worker in a community facility for people with physical and learning disabilities. Jack started by doing some agency shifts and found that he really enjoyed the work and felt it was more socially meaningful than anything he had done previously.

Along the way, he has acquired a partner and a small child so his decision to enter nurse training is a bit of a short-term sacrifice, but he and his partner have talked it through. He hopes it will lead to a fulfilling long-term career and a good means of supporting his family.

Jack is enjoying the teaching and mixing with other like-minded students on his course. He has been on a couple of placements. These have gone well but have also served to reinforce the idea that there is much to be done to achieve more equality and respect for people with learning disabilities. He is very aware of the tendency for people to ignore the person with a disability and instead address the carer.

Visit the Values Exchange website at http://sagecomms.vxcommunity.com for a broader discussion on this Student story.

Communication may be commonly assumed to be a simple two-way exchange of information. However, it is much more than that and in nursing and midwifery, for much of the time, it is necessary to have communication that demonstrates compassion where one 'must be receptive to another's communication' and 'put him/herself in the other's place' (Reynolds, 2005). Patients and service users can be extremely anxious as to what might lie ahead. The impact of a kind and compassionate approach should never be underestimated, as Patient story 1.1, taken from Patientopinion.org/, demonstrates. The Patient Opinion website has been operational in the UK for over 10 years and provides real-time feedback to healthcare services (patientopinion.org.uk).

Patient story 1.1: Gratitude

I honestly can't thank the nurses and doctors at ***** unit enough for their care and compassion during my visit. I have luckily never had a stay in hospital before this visit so I had been initially apprehensive but the nurses soon eased my worries when I entered the ward. The staff were very attentive, efficient and friendly. Even though I quite suddenly required more treatment than I had initially expected, I felt very reassured by the nurses and doctors throughout the whole experience. If it hadn't been for their professionalism and compassion, I would have felt frightened by the change in the situation. They kept me informed about everything that was going to happen and treated me with exceptional kindness. There was one nurse in particular (I am sorry I can't remember her name) who was with me throughout and was absolutely fantastic, thank you! (www.patientopinion.org.uk/, 2016)

This is the type of patient feedback that everyone wants to hear. Traditionally, the nursing profession has been commonly assumed to contain people who can communicate and possess 'caring' and 'compassionate' characteristics. Indeed, it is deemed mandatory by the national governing bodies that candidates for entry to the profession exhibit these characteristics at the recruitment stage (Bryson and Jones, 2013). Despite these gatekeeping efforts, however, recent scandals such as The Francis Report (Francis, 2010, 2013) and the inquiry into Winterbourne View (Bubb, 2014) have revealed a troubling paradox wherein those within an ostensibly 'caring' profession have failed to exhibit such fundamental characteristics of care and benevolence to devastating effect for patients and their carers. Investigations into these scandals repeatedly identified compassionate, collaborative and effective communication as severely lacking.

The following extracts are taken from two reports produced by Sir Robert Francis at the request of health ministers following complaints by relatives of service users at the Mid Staffordshire NHS Foundation Trust.

Patient story 1.2: The Mid Staffordshire care scandal

Following a fall the patient was admitted to Stafford Hospital. When the patient requested a bedpan he was told by the nurse to soil himself as she was too busy to help. (Francis, 2010, p. 6)

The first inquiry heard harrowing personal stories from patients and patients' families about the appalling care received at the Trust. On many occasions, the accounts received related to basic elements of care and the quality of the patient experience. These included cases where: Patients were left in excrement in soiled bed clothes for lengthy periods; Assistance was not provided with feeding for patients who could not eat without help; Water was left out of reach; In spite of persistent requests for help, patients were not assisted in their toileting; Wards and toilet facilities were left in a filthy condition; Privacy and dignity, even in death, were denied; Triage in A&E was undertaken by untrained staff; Staff treated patients and those close to them with what appeared to be callous indifference. (Francis, 2013, p. 25)

The press, politicians and organisations representing service users have rightly expressed outrage at this state of affairs and demanded change (www.patients-association.com). Such scandals of poor health and social care, however, are not unique to this decade. Vulnerable service users have been the recipients of neglect and even abuse over many years. Timmins (2012) points out that the traditional method of funding healthcare used to rely on a little more funding than the previous year, plus extra to cover an inevitable scandal. Although exemplary care is delivered by many professionals, at the same time, others lose the capacity to maintain and sustain a compassionate approach. Behaviours demonstrating poor communication, uncompassionate care and disinterest in collaborative relationships with patients and service users have not only been an endemic feature of health and social care, they are also almost considered par for the course.

Lack of compassion is a recurring theme in many reports of poor healthcare. For the recipient, compassion goes hand in hand with good communication. There are various definitions of compassion, including sympathy, pity, and a desire to help or alleviate suffering

(Baughan and Smith, 2013). However, we would suggest that the quality of empathy – a recognition of others' emotions, the ability to see the situation from their perspective – is more useful for the professional demonstration of compassion in contemporary times (Dinkins, 2011). Empathy, like communication, may be assumed to be intrinsic to human nature, however the effective demonstration and maintenance of empathy are not so simple.

The concept of 'burnout' for professionals in caring work is well known and documented in the literature. Burnout and desensitisation are real risks which can lead to a high level of breakdown in communication (Personal communication with year 3 nursing students, 2014). Burnout is associated with emotional blunting and uncaring attitudes towards service users (Zhang et al., 2014). It is widely acknowledged that professionals in health and social care need to be open to and attend to their own emotions to prevent 'compassion fatigue' and burnout (Baughan and Smith, 2013, p. 77). (This concept will be revisited in some depth in future chapters, alongside techniques to enable you to avoid burnout and preserve an empathic and compassionate approach.)

Communication problems have remained one of the most common sources of complaint in health services in the UK and in other countries. Reader et al. (2014, p. 685) found that complaints about problematic communication and poor staff–patient relationships 'were almost equal' in number to those about the quality of clinical care. The quotations in Patient story 1.3 have been taken from recent postings on the UK Patientopinion. org/ website. These statements illustrate the heightened emotions and anxieties of health service users and carers and how this experience is either ameliorated or worsened by communication with health professionals.

Patient story 1.3: Positive and negative communication

A desperately worrying and devastating time for us, as my father was very poorly and vulnerable. The doctor showed exceptional medical care and compassion to helping my father get the best possible care he could.

I was treated with respect from the time I arrived. It made such a difference to have someone take the time to undertake an examination and explain the findings and treatment plan without trying to rush you through.

In this instance I am disgusted by the lack of compassion, empathy and help shown primarily towards my mother but also to me ... To sum up: the care of my 95-year-old father who has dementia lacked dignity or any sense of urgency that any person of any age should expect.

A hospital was supposed to be a place to feel safe and cared for but not in this case. Summary – lack of compassion and care, low numbers of qualified staff, light left on in wards at night and very noisy talking laughing staff at nursing stations at night.

(www.patientopinion.org.uk/, 2014)

These quotations describe people from the same professions but with very differing presentations to patients. In order to safeguard against such examples of poor communication in the delivery of healthcare, it is crucial to consider how healthcare professionals who seemingly start out with positive intentions may intentionally or unintentionally end up exhibiting negative attitudes and behaviours towards those for whom they are supposed to care. Communicative behaviour is the outward expression of health professionals' internal attitudes and values (Gault et al., 2013). Consequently, it is necessary to examine the ethical values underpinning and enabling positive attitudes and behaviours in caring for others.

Respect and dignity

How will you ensure that your practice demonstrates respect and preserves dignity?

The Nursing and Midwifery code of conduct in the UK explicitly states that 'you must treat people as individuals and respect their dignity' (NMC, 2015, p. 4). Service user comments emphasise the importance of being respected and not treated in an undignified manner. Many healthcare procedures have the capacity for great indignity. Again, Patientopinion. org/ (2015) illustrates how healthcare staff can minimise the potential indignity by communicating respect and empathy or, alternatively, worsen the experience.

Patient story 1.4: Dignity and respect

Due to the nature of the tests and procedures it could have been embarrassing and unpleasant but everyone was so nice and accommodating I almost forgot where I was! ... Treated with dignity and care for a potentially embarrassing investigation.

I'm embarrassed talking about my condition, at the best of times. But to be in the hands of someone whom I thought would have been a professional; I have been left feeling degraded, and a little violated at the lack of respect and dignity I was shown.

(www.patientopinion.org.uk/, 2015)

Clearly, as illustrated by the quotations in Patient story 1.4, it is possible to be careless in communication and to leave the service user feeling humiliated. Wainwright and Gallagher (2008) discuss how easily (and unthinkingly) professionals may reinforce the experience of disrespect, through simple and repeated acts of carelessness. Becoming a patient or health service user almost always involves dependence on the healthcare practitioner, with considerable scope for violation of privacy. Codes of conduct now emphasise the need for nurses and midwives to understand the 'trust and privilege inherent in the relationship between nurses and people receiving care' (Nursing and Midwifery Board of Australia, 2008, p. 1), and their obligation to minimise the power imbalance between patient and professional.

These complex understandings and interactions can appear a challenging task. However, nurses and midwives can develop both intellectual interpretations and practical behaviours relating to respect and dignity with the aid of relevant theory. Respect is defined as 'to hold in high regard; to show consideration for others' (Mosby, 2012). Fraser and Honneth's (2003) theory of recognition focuses on respect and helps in understanding how feeling disrespected (as in the patientopinion.org/ statement above) is deeply wounding. He argues that a lack of respect or disrespect is damaging, interfering with our existing sense of identity acquired through years of interaction with others. To find oneself denied respect in any situation is an assault on identity and self-esteem. The use of inappropriate verbal and non-verbal responses to someone attempting to talk about their 'embarrassing' condition communicates disrespect to that person.

Nordenfelt discusses 'dignity of identity' (2009, p. xiii). This type of dignity underpins respect for human rights and relates to the value or worth people have purely on the basis of their being human and regardless of ethnicity, social class, gender or sexual orientation. The Royal College of Nursing (2008) also affirms that dignity is associated with identity and feelings of self-worth or how 'people feel, think and behave in relation to the worth or value of themselves'. Gallagher (2004) provides an example of an elderly person presented with a cup of tea minus a saucer. Although the young nurse seemed oblivious to the fact, the older woman, due to her age, class and value system, felt that she had been insulted. She believed that being given tea without a saucer indicated a lack of respect for her identity and thus was an affront to her dignity.

One of the ways in which we demonstrate respect is in our willingness (or lack of it) to work co-operatively with others. The NMC code of conduct also states that 'you must work in partnership with people to make sure you deliver care effectively' (Nursing and Midwifery Council, 2015, p. 5). It might be assumed that as healthcare practitioners we automatically include the service user in decision making and communication about their care. Conversely, collaborative communication is a complex skill but one that is essential not only in healthcare but also in modern life generally. As Sennett (2012) notes, in his book *Together*, most of us exist as social animals within societies, with many interdependencies. Few, if any, can manage to get through life without interaction with others. Co-operation and communication between humans are necessary to both avoid conflict and make progress. However, as demonstrated by history, the ability to communicate and co-operate with one another has often been in short supply. Humans, throughout history, have tended towards tribalism or the tendency to feel solidarity only with those perceived as similar to themselves. Tribalism is dangerous in contemporary life and, as Sennett notes (2012, p. 3), 'in the form of nationalism, destroyed Europe during the first half of the twentieth century'. Whereas tribalism might have been helpful historically in very simple societies, it becomes a problem in current, complex societies where the ability to communicate collaboratively with those who differ from ourselves is essential (Sennett, 2012).

Healthcare professionals exist like everyone else within society, have been socialised within that society and are likely to enter healthcare education holding the values with which they have grown up. Here, again, communicative collaboration is an example of a task that may look simple on the outside but is actually an intricate endeavour. Therefore, an understanding and examination of our capacity to truly collaborate versus our tendency towards tribal behaviour are required. Are healthcare workers likely to hold judgemental attitudes towards those dissimilar to themselves? Does the health professional really want to work collaboratively with the service user or do they actually wish to tell the service user how to behave?

CRITICAL THINKING EXERCISE 1.1
———————— CONSIDER THE FOLLOWING SCENARIOS ————————
AND EXPLORE YOUR RESPONSE

You are on placement in a surgical ward in a large general hospital. A fellow student seems to make remarks that you feel are judgemental when referring to patients. He says things like 'Asian people do this' or 'gay people are known to do that'. Should we accept this behaviour from another student? Should you act on this and, if so, how?

You are on placement in a community mental health team. One of the service users tells you and your mentor that she is not taking her medication as prescribed. She has a history of relapse when she fails to take medication. She says it makes her drowsy and interferes with her ability to look after her children. What would be your response?

The centrality and complexity of communication in the therapeutic relationship

Do you think that communication comes naturally and that you will easily build therapeutic relationships?

Building therapeutic relationships and demonstrating effective healthcare communication are complex skills, based on positive professional values and ethical practice (Seago, 2008). It is recognised that students in nursing and midwifery need to develop highly sophisticated communication skills to provide compassionate care to the people they look after (NMC, 2010). Student contributors to this book reported that they often start their learning programme feeling that they already know how to communicate and questioned the value of this part of the course. Seago (2008) and Happell (2009) also support this perspective, emphasising that people generally underestimate the complexity of healthcare communication. On commencing modules in communication skills, students report an increasing awareness of the importance, and difficulty, of this area of skill development. This includes how to break bad news, how to communicate with relatives, how to ensure someone has understood important information, how to work with the person to develop collaborative plans to improve health (rather than just 'telling' someone what to do), how to deal with colleagues who do not communicate in the best way with their patients, how to communicate new ideas about good practice and influence change – all these and more are communication challenges for students.

The therapeutic relationship will be discussed at length throughout the book but it requires some brief exploration at this point. 'Therapeutic' is considered to be an essential element in healthcare relationships but also a term much used and possibly abused in healthcare. The dictionary defines 'therapeutic' as 'the art of healing' or 'concerned with the remedial treatment of disease' (OED, OUP, 2003, p. 455). It can take many forms such as curative, preventative, supportive or palliative. Chambers (2005, p. 302) notes that 'therapeutic relationships … can be taken for granted', yet they are rarely explored or challenged in any meaningful manner. Garwood-Gowers et al. (2005) argue that the term itself is problematic as there is little consensus on what therapeutic means. There has been a tendency to be content with the term 'therapeutic' meaning whatever the particular practitioner wishes it to mean. Therefore, if the practitioner has convinced themself that what they do is 'therapeutic', the service user is simply expected to agree.

It is, therefore, necessary to explore the therapeutic relationship rather than assume we must be therapeutic simply because we wear the uniform. Dzopia and Ahern (2009) explore the factors that make a relationship therapeutic in character. Qualities of warmth, genuineness, not being judgemental and conveying understanding are cited but, as they acknowledge, these can be difficult to define. Displaying the communicative behaviours of relating to the patient as a person, being available and signalling a desire to help are perceived as therapeutic by patients (Williams and Irurita, 2004). Yet, too often, it is assumed that these values and skills are easily acquired or even intrinsic to human nature.

CRITICAL THINKING EXERCISE 1.2
CONSIDER THE STATEMENTS BELOW
AND RESPOND TO EACH

The audience does not play a role in communication.

People who speak the same language do not have a problem with communication.

Speaking directly is universally acceptable.

The more words used in communicating, the better.

It is the speaker's job to make me understand.

Communication is an inborn talent – either you have it or you don't.

Non-verbal signals are universally understood.

Silence is not feedback.

Communication means giving information.

Visit the Values Exchange website at http://sagecomms.vxcommunity.com to develop your critical thinking skills and debate your thoughts and decisions.

Student contributors to this book described their 'worst fears' on commencing their first early practice placements. Although younger students felt anxious at the prospect of providing adequate communicative support to older patients, more mature students suggested they had even more to fear. One of these described experiences where staff and patients would assume that she had abilities well beyond her sphere of competence as a first-year student. Both groups of students agreed that they experienced feelings of fear and embarrassment when confronted with difficult communicative situations on placement (Student focus group, 2013).

Student story 1.3: 'Your worst fear'

You are a first-year student on a placement on a hospital ward. You have been working here for three weeks and have settled into the demands of the placement with commitment and enthusiasm. As a result of your dedication, you are popular amongst the clientele, and have built positive therapeutic relationships with all of them. Your mentor is pleased with your

(Continued)

(Continued)

progress, and the staff team tell you that you are the kind of person that they would like to employ once you qualify.

'Ruth' was admitted during your second week. She is a 24-year-old woman with whom you feel you have a close professional relationship. She has a partner and two small children and they all clearly love each other very much. You cannot help but be touched by this, and by the deep affection Ruth shows to both her children (who are 2 and 3 years old), as well as her partner. They are also very fond of you, and often talk about you and their gratitude for your good care of Ruth.

There was some mystery surrounding Ruth's admission, and so she was admitted for tests, of which she has now undertaken many. Her results are now due.

You arrive for your shift today, and your mentor says that Ruth has asked to see you specifically, although she doesn't know why. Approaching Ruth, she asks you for a 'very large favour' and then bursts into tears. She explains that her results have revealed that she has a very rare form of an especially aggressive cancer, and it is now developed to such a stage that there is nothing that can be done except palliative care; the consultant has told her that she has about 10–20 days left.

Ruth is understandably devastated, particularly as she had no inkling that she was terminally ill. She now feels horribly guilty for making light and joking with the children about being ill, as she assumed she'd be home in no time. Her partner doesn't know as yet, and she thinks that he won't cope with the terrible news well at all, as he's 'super sensitive'.

Because of all this, Ruth doesn't believe that either she or her partner are the best people to explain the situation to their children, and the favour she is asking is for you to sit down and do this for them instead. She says she knows it's a huge thing to ask, but she has noticed how kind, clever and professional you are...

- What would you do?
- How would you feel?
- What would you say?
- What would you be telling yourself?

This is a frightening prospect and unlikely to happen on your early placements but it does describe the worst imaginings of student nurses who reflect on the initial stages of their course. The scenario above represents a situation that is potentially challenging to the novice practitioner. However, this is not designed to scare students off before they start but to illustrate the sensitive context of the world of healthcare communication. In order to be communicatively and ethically competent, the following chapters within this book will enable you to reflect and develop coping and communicative skills for scenarios such as this.

Critical debate 1.1: The good communicator

Can compassion and good communication be learned or are these qualities that one is born with?
    If these can be learned, what is the best method?
    If you think that compassion and good communicative skills are qualities we are born with, what should we do about colleagues who seem to lack them?

Conclusion

To conclude, communication within the therapeutic relationship is a complex task and there are too many instances where it has gone badly wrong. Nevertheless, the current cries of outrage at failures in compassionate care and communication are not new but a persistent feature in some areas of healthcare. In many cases, the inability of nurses and midwives to care for their own emotional wellbeing results in poor care for service users. There is a tendency to assume that good communication skills and a compassionate nature simply come with the job. We argue that this is a dangerous assumption. Effective and empathic communication can be enhanced by an appreciation of the ethical and theoretical understanding underpinning complex but essential communication skills. Practitioners need to learn how to look after their own emotions and to recognise emotion in others alongside skill acquisition. The following chapters will break these elements into their constituent parts and enable the learner to develop emotionally, theoretically and practically.

Further suggested activity

Explore patient websites/social media outlets. What are they saying about health services? What are their most persistent complaints? Try the following websites:

Hello my name is home page – www.hellomynameis.org.uk – or #hellomynameis campaign on Twitter
Patient Opinion home page – www.patientopinion.org.uk/
The Patients Association home page – www.patients-association.com

To access further resources related to this chapter, visit the Values Exchange website at http:// sagecomms.vxcommunity.com

References

Baughan, J. and Smith, A. (2013) *Compassion, Caring and Communication*, 2nd edn. London: Pearson Education.

Bryson, T. and Jones, L. (2013) *Mental Health Nursing Recruitment and Selection.* London: Health Education North West London, Health Education North East and Central London and Health Education South London.

Bubb, S. (2014) *Winterbourne View: Time for Change.* Transforming Care and Commissioning Group. Available at: www.england.nhs.uk/wp-content/uploads/2014/11/transforming-commissioning-services.pdf (accessed 24 March 2016).

Chambers, M. (2005) 'A concept analysis of therapeutic relationships', in J. Cutcliffe and H. McKenna (eds), *The Essential Concepts of Nursing.* Edinburgh: Elsevier. pp. 301–16.

Dinkins, C. (2011) 'Ethics: beyond patient care – practicing empathy in the workplace', *Online Journal of Issues in Nursing*, 16(2).

Dzopia, F. and Ahern, K. (2009) 'What makes a quality therapeutic relationship in psychiatric/ mental health nursing: a review of the literature', *The Internet Journal of Advanced Nursing*, 10(1): 8–12.

Francis, R. (2010) *Independent Inquiry into Care provided by Mid Staffordshire NHS Foundation Trust January 2005 – March 2009.* London: The Stationery Office.

Francis, R. (2013) *The Mid Staffordshire NHS Foundation Trust Public Inquiry.* London: The Stationery Office.

Fraser, N. and Honneth, A. (2003) *Redistribution or Recognition: A Political-Philosophical Exchange*. London: Verso.

Gallagher A. (2004) 'Dignity and respect for dignity: two key health professional values – implications for nursing practice', *Nursing Ethics*, 11(6): 587–99.

Garwood-Gowers, A., Tingle, J. and Wheat, K. (2005) *Contemporary Issues in Healthcare Law and Ethics*. Oxford: Elsevier.

Gault, I., Chambers, M. and Gallagher, A. (2013) 'Perspectives on medicine adherence in service users and carers with experience of legally sanctioned detention and medication: a qualitative study', *Patient Preference and Adherence*, 8 August, 7: 787–99.

Happell, B. (2009) 'Influencing undergraduate nursing students' attitudes toward mental health nursing: acknowledging the role of theory', *Issues in Mental Health Nursing*, 30(1): 39–46.

Mosby (2012) *Mosby Medical Dictionary*, 9th edition. Bethesda, MD: Mosby.

Nordenfelt, L. (ed.) (2009) *Dignity in Care for Older People*. Oxford: Wiley Blackwell.

Nursing and Midwifery Board of Australia (2008) *Code of Professional Conduct*. Melbourne: National Midwifery Board of Australia.

Nursing and Midwifery Council (NMC) England (2010) *Standards for Pre-registration Nursing*. London: NMC.

Nursing and Midwifery Council (NMC) (2015) *Code of Conduct*. London: NMC.

OUP (2003) *Oxford English Dictionary*, 2nd edn. Oxford: Oxford University Press.

Reader, T., Gillespie, A. and Roberts, J. (2014) 'Patient complaints in healthcare systems: a systematic review and coding taxonomy', *BMJ Quality & Safety*, 23(8): 678–689.

Reynolds, W. (2005) 'The concept of empathy', in J. Cutcliffe and H. McKenna (eds), *The Essential Concepts of Nursing*. Edinburgh: Elsevier. pp. 93–108.

Royal College of Nursing (RCN) (2008) *Definition of Dignity*. Available at www.rcn.org.uk/clinical-topics/nutrition-and-hydration/current-work/dignity, accessed 7 December 2015.

Seago, J. (2008) 'Professional communication patient safety and quality', in *An Evidence-Based Handbook for Nurses: Vol. 2*. New York: Pearson. pp. 242–7.

Sennett, R. (2012) *Together: The Rituals, Pleasures and Politics of Co-operation*. London: Allen Lane.

Timmins, N. (2012) *Never Again: The Story of the Health and Social Care Act 2012*. London: The Kings Fund.

Wainwright, P. and Gallagher, A. (2008) 'On different types of dignity in nursing care: a critique of Nordenfelt', *Nursing Philosophy*, 9: 46–54.

Williams, A.M. and Irurita, V.F. (2004) 'Therapeutic and non-therapeutic interpersonal interactions: the patient's perspective', *Journal of Clinical Nursing*, 13: 806–815.

Zhang, X., Huang, D. and Guan, P. (2014) 'Job burnout among critical care nurses from 14 adult intensive care units in northeastern China: a cross-sectional survey', *British Medical Journal: BMJ Open*, 4(6): e004813.

2

Essential Communication Skills: Building Blocks for Good Communication

Jean Shapcott and Iris Gault

By the end of this chapter, you will have developed an understanding of:

- verbal, non-verbal and written communication: listening, questioning, record keeping, electronic prescribing
- professional communication, social and professional media, and professional identity
- the use of reflection on practice.

Don't forget to visit the Values Exchange website at http://sagecomms.vxcommunity.com for extra practice and revision activities.

• •

Introduction

Chapter 2 will initially consider the basic behavioural building blocks for good communication: verbal and non-verbal skills, how to properly listen, how to effectively use questions and how to handle 21st-century electronic forms of communication. These are essential tools for nursing, yet not always adequately undertaken. It will then go on to explore how professional identity influences professional communication. The advantages and potential pitfalls of professional and social media are explored. Finally, we consider how reflection on practice can enhance communication and collaboration. Reflection is an important component of professional practice and one to which we return at points throughout the book.

Non-verbal, verbal and written communication: listening, questioning, record keeping, electronic prescribing

Student story 2.1: Josh

Josh is a first-year mental health nursing student. He is 21, and he couldn't quite decide what to do when he finished school with three middling A levels. He took a gap year with the original intention of making up his mind what degree to do whilst enjoying himself in the sun. However, when he got back, he found that he still hadn't decided what to do. His parents started to get annoyed at him for drifting and strongly suggested he get some employment. His mother worked as an administrator at the local psychiatric hospital and managed to get him an interview for a healthcare assistant post in the forensic unit. He got the job and, much to his surprise, found that he enjoyed the work. He got on well with the staff and most of the service users. He was initially a bit apprehensive at the thought of working with offenders but settled into the work well. Some of the nurses could talk with and listen to the service users but Jack and most of the other healthcare assistants felt that they needed to be 'firm but fair'. The hospital has now offered to sponsor him to do his nurse education and he is a few weeks into his first year. He still has contact with a nominated mentor at the hospital, who has told him he will need to work on his communication skills, but Josh thinks he has already proved he can communicate.

We will define the basic elements of communication and ask some questions about their effectiveness in healthcare. Whether communication is voluntary or involuntary, it exists within all human beings and is fundamental to human life (McCabe and Timmins, 2006). Communication is a two-way process and a complex interaction during which information passes between individuals. It is cyclical in nature, allowing a message to be sent and received, following which there will be either confirmation of receipt of the information or interpretation of the interaction as successful or otherwise.

A number of communication theorists will be referred to throughout the book but it is to Noam Chomsky (1979) that we turn at this point. He suggests that language is an innate faculty and that people are born with a set of rules about language in their heads. Despite language being a complex system, most children acquire language effortlessly and in a relatively short time without any formal teaching. It is commonly believed that children learn language through mimicry, but Chomsky would argue that language acquisition involves very little imitation, if any. He also indicated that reinforcement – the use of correction and reward – plays little role in the active process of language acquisition during which children often say things that they have never heard from adults. Chomsky concluded that infants are born with a 'language acquisition device' and that exposure to language is all that is needed for a child to discover the system of language.

However, professional communication differs from everyday communication and requires more than exposure to the professional setting. Effective communication skills are essential within nursing and are often seen as one of the main skills necessary for nurses to support patients and their families (Dougherty and Lister, 2011). The provision of high-quality holistic care requires good communication to ensure that the wellbeing of the patient remains at the forefront of care and that patients and their families receive the information they require to participate in their own care according to their individual preference. It is therefore crucial that nurses use the full range of communication skills at their disposal, whilst ensuring that the intentions of any nurse–patient interaction are clear.

There are two forms of communication: verbal and non-verbal. Verbal communication involves the use of either the spoken or written word. Generally, people feel they are competent speakers. Students involved in feeding back on course content reported feeling mildly insulted on hearing they must learn basic communication skills, claiming: 'we already know how to speak and communicate otherwise we wouldn't have got through the interview' (Focus group, 2013). Nevertheless, problems with communication account for large numbers of complaints about the health service (Parliamentary and Health Service Ombudsman, 2011). Much of this is due to problematic written and verbal communication.

CRITICAL THINKING EXERCISE 2.1
WHY WON'T PATIENTS DO WHAT WE SAY?

Why do so many patients report that they do not understand what was said to them?

Soon after cardiac health problems, 34% stopped taking Aspirin, in the longer term 45% stopped Beta blockers, and after two years only 40% were still taking prescribed statins (Ho et al., 2009).

There may be many factors involved but research shows that patients and service users do not receive the message where they perceive healthcare professionals to be less than interested in them (Clyne et al., 2007; Gault, 2009). In addition, factors such as culture, language, tone of voice, speech rate and accent will influence the effectiveness of the spoken word, as may a sensory impairment in a patient. It is important to speak clearly and concisely and ensure that what is being said actually reflects what the speaker intends to say to ensure that the receiver understands the message (Kozier et al., 2012). The use of jargon should be avoided as it has the potential to increase patient anxiety.

Paralinguistics, or non-verbal communication, also influences the message. This includes all of the actions that accompany speech (Sikorski, 2012). Non-verbal communication (NVC) is often referred to as 'body language', although the two terms are not necessarily interchangeable. It is a very powerful medium for communication. NVC includes physical appearance, gesture, eye contact, facial expression and touch. Physical appearance is important as it creates an immediate impact. For example, on first meeting a nurse, many patients are influenced by whether or not that nurse appears professional. Often, communication occurs through the overall effect of a number of aspects of NVC, for example a gesture may be only a hand movement, but when combined with limited eye contact it might be interpreted as disinterest or guilt. Touch, whilst an important element of NVC which conveys empathy, support, presence and caring, must be utilised carefully as it can easily be misconstrued.

Schmidt Bunkers (2010) explores how listening and questioning can demonstrate that the professional is interested in and focused on the patient. Too often, patients are left feeling that they have not been heard. Active listening is a primary source of communication for nurses. What patients say about themselves is very important and, in order to be an active listener, nurses need to be engaged in receiving and decoding the messages that patients send. This involves not only listening to the verbal content of the message, but also observing the patient's non-verbal communication and integrating this information in assessing their current emotional state. Nurses listen to a patient with two purposes in mind – to comprehend the message and to evaluate its meaning. As a consequence of active listening, nurses are able to paraphrase (summarise and repeat back) the content of a patient's message in different ways throughout the interaction, thus ensuring they have received the message accurately, especially in very intense conversations (Montague et al., 2013).

The appropriate use of questions complements active listening in nurse–patient interactions. There are many forms of questions which can lead the interaction in distinctive directions and provide diverse responses. Closed questions are directive in nature and are driven by the needs of the nurse for information. Consequently, they have a specific fact-finding purpose and can be quickly answered with one word or very short responses. An example might be: 'Do you live at 10, The Avenue?' to which the patient can only respond 'Yes' or 'No'. Closed questions have their place, but they do not explore the patient's agenda because their answer and involvement in the communication process are restricted. When a nurse wishes to elicit a patient's perceptions, ideas and feelings, open questions invite them into the conversation at a more participative level, since they provide opportunities to talk freely about their experiences, things that interest them and their concerns (Lambert, 2012). Schmidt Bunkers (2010) also adds that 'why' questions should be avoided as these can sound accusatory.

CRITICAL THINKING EXERCISE 2.2
DO YOU LISTEN?

- Make a written record of all the discussions that you have today.
- For each discussion, ask yourself the following questions: What was the subject under discussion? Who talked most? Did I learn anything that I didn't already know?
- Do this for at least three discussions to find out your current level of listening skills.

Written communication, record keeping, electronic record keeping and prescribing

Nurses are required to use written communication when accurately documenting the care given to a patient. Nursing notes, which are increasingly being recorded electronically, are legal documents and can be produced in court as evidence. An incomplete or insufficient record can lead the court to determine that the care given to a patient was not of a reasonable standard, particularly since many months or years may have elapsed before a case comes to court. Documentation must be completed contemporaneously and should be specific, factual, accurate, measurable, written in standardised medical or English terminology, avoiding jargon and abbreviations and tailored to the unique characteristics of each individual and their care (Kozier et al., 2012). Severe failure can result in losing the right to practise:

As a member of the wider health care team, the health care assistant (HCA), assistant practitioner (AP) or nursing student takes personal accountability for good record keeping. They must keep clear, accurate and timely records of the care they provide to their patients to support communication, continuity and decision making. (www.rcn.org)

CRITICAL THINKING EXERCISE 2.3
DOCUMENTATION

On your clinical placements, undertake an exercise whereby you look at documentation completed by a range of nurses – qualified and nursing students – and measure this against the following criteria. Is it:

* specific?
* factual?
* accurate?
* measurable?
* written in standardised medical or English terminology, avoiding jargon and abbreviations?
* tailored to the unique characteristics of each individual and their care?
* written in a way that could enable someone to determine the care a patient had received from the report documented?

Twenty-first century healthcare providers are moving to many forms of electronic communication including e-prescribing. Tolley (2012) considers an ideal world where record keeping would be centralised, accessible, and where all medication miscommunication would be a thing of the past. Cornford et al. (2009, p. 8) point out that 'prescribing errors occur in 1.5–9.2% of medication orders written for hospital inpatients, dispensing errors are identified in 0.02% of dispensed items, medication administration errors occur in 3.0–8.0% of non-intravenous doses and about 50% of all intravenous doses'.

Quereshi et al. (2015) found that although not perfect, e-prescribing substantially reduced error and healthcare costs. Electronic communication is not an issue simply for those doctors and nurses who are prescribers but for all staff involved in caring for patients and in medication administration. In future, it is expected that all healthcare providers will be moving to forms of electronic communication, and consequently it is important that student and qualified healthcare staff are prepared for this change.

Professional communication, professional identity, and social and professional media
The use of professional and social media

Communication is now very different from that of 20 years ago. In the 21st century, the use of social and professional media has proliferated. Chin (2012) points out that by 2011, Ofcom calculated that 48% of adults used social and professional media regularly.

There are numerous sites and as Chin notes, many, including Twitter, can provide excellent opportunities for professional-to-professional communication. Wren (2012) also notes that use of social media can be a very positive method of communication in healthcare. If used responsibly and appropriately, these can offer several benefits for nurses, midwives and students. They include:

- building and maintaining professional relationships
- establishing or accessing nursing and midwifery support networks and being able to discuss specific issues, interests, research and clinical experiences with other healthcare professionals globally
- being able to access resources for continuing professional development (CPD).

However, students may jeopardise their ability to join the Nursing and Midwifery Council register, if they act in any way that is unprofessional or unlawful on social media, including (but not limited to):

- 'sharing confidential information inappropriately
- posting pictures of patients and people receiving care without their consent
- posting inappropriate comments about patients
- bullying, intimidating or exploiting people
- building or pursuing relationships with patients or service users
- stealing personal information or using someone else's identity
- encouraging violence or self-harm
- inciting hatred or discrimination'. (Nursing and Midwifery Council, 2015, p. 3)

It is therefore essential that nurses remain professional whenever they use professional and social media, which includes not accepting patients or family members as friends on any networking site, not posting pictures of patients or their families, and being very careful what they say about where they work or what their work involves:

> Protect your professionalism and your reputation. If you are unsure whether something you post online could compromise your professionalism or your reputation, you should think about what the information means for you in practice and how it affects your responsibility to keep to the Code. It is important to consider who and what you associate with on social media. For example, acknowledging someone else's post can imply that you endorse or support their point of view. You should consider the possibility of other people mentioning you in inappropriate posts. If you have used social media for a number of years, it is important to consider, in relation to the Code, what you have posted online in the past. (Nursing and Midwifery Council, 2015, p. 8)

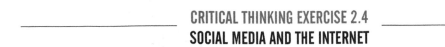

CRITICAL THINKING EXERCISE 2.4
SOCIAL MEDIA AND THE INTERNET

Are there any pictures on social media that could reflect badly on your professional image?
  If you were someone else looking at these pictures, what would you think about that person?

 Visit the Values Exchange website at http://sagecomms.vxcommunity.com to develop your critical thinking skills and debate your thoughts and decisions.

Professional identity

Just as it is important that nurses and midwives are communicatively competent and compassionate, it is necessary to consider how professional identity influences communication. Nursing identity has evolved to that of a graduate profession, and this means that the underlying rationale and knowledge base are becoming more sophisticated and complex. Professional communication is integral to any professional identity and particularly pertinent at this time. Public confidence in health professionals has been adversely affected by the scandals of indifferent or even cruel behaviour in healthcare settings. Health professionals must communicate that they are practising ethically and effectively (McKewan and Harris, 2010).

To communicate effectively, nurses and midwives need to develop confident and positive professional identities. Developing and being socialised into this identity is a complex process that requires high levels of *personal* self-awareness and a willingness to engage and empathise with others, even in the most difficult of circumstances … however, we suspect you knew that already.

CRITICAL THINKING EXERCISE 2.5
PERSONAL AND PROFESSIONAL IDENTITY

- Why is there this emphasis on the 'personal' when you are learning to be a professional?
- How confident are you in your professional identity?

Think about these questions and write down honest answers.

Johnson et al. (2012, p. 562) assert that 'A positive and flexible professional identity is critical for nurses to function at a high level and benefits not only nurses themselves, but also patients and other healthcare workers'. They note that although some might enter the profession with innate confidence and high self-esteem, most people develop their self-identity through interaction and reflection on that interaction with others.

Students in healthcare often report that they lack confidence both personally and professionally, in the early stages of their courses. Becoming a professional helps to build confidence and reflection is key to developing your professional identity. All subject areas studied including communication will require you to develop your ability to reflect on your learning and understanding in order to put these theories into practice. Reflection is defined as 'a generic term for those intellectual and affective activities in which individuals engage to explore their experiences in order to lead to a new understanding and appreciation' (Boud, 1983, p. 19, cited in Mann et al., 2009, p. 597).

Reflective learning (through use of personal experience and knowledge) is now a key part of training for nurses and other professionals in health and social care. Reflective practice means observing our interactions with others, and then analysing our thoughts, feelings and behaviours using relevant knowledge/theory. It is an ongoing process that you will continue throughout the length of your career (Bulman and Shutz, 2013). Okuda and Fukada's (2014) study of nursing students involved in reflective dialogue indicated that this process can help students define and refine their professional identities. Participants first self-reflected on their practice and then discussed their reflection with others: 'The thoughts that guide nurses' work and the ability to discover meaning and significance in work while questioning oneself are matters that allow professionals to play their roles well' (2014, p. 22).

CRITICAL THINKING EXERCISE 2.6
WHO ARE YOU?

What are your reflections about yourself? How does your personal identity affect your professional identity?

- What is your preferred method of communication – written/spoken? Do you communicate quietly or with lots of gesticulation?
- How comfortable are you with space? Do you touch and hug easily?
- Are you affiliated with any social/religious/cultural/sporting/leisure groups?
- Do you prefer to spend time on your own or with close family?
- Do you believe that we control our own destiny or that fate controls our lives?

Reflecting on or looking back at both your core beliefs and your performance in practice is helpful in working towards a positive professional identity. This allows for the ability to assess and appraise performance in the light of knowledge about effective communication and to build on and improve your practice.

The use of reflection on practice

We now invite you to reflect on your own practice and consider your communicative and collaborative abilities. Ghaye (2010) supports the point that how people feel affects thinking and that, in turn, influences what we do. He argues that reflection allows us to structure and organise those feelings and thoughts to improve action or future practice. He cites Schön (1983) as one of the most important writers on reflective practice. Schön distinguished reflection in action from reflection on practice. In action means thinking on your feet or responding immediately. This will be a major part of your communicative practice. However, reflecting on your practice at a later point is essential for developing and improving your communication skills. The use of reflective models or cycles can enable a structured and organised evaluation of practice, plus a plan to strengthen future communication.

Ghaye (2010) argues that it is necessary to approach reflection from a positive perspective. Often, we attempt to improve by examining deficits but he points out that a deficit-based approach often ends up with deficit-based answers! This links with previous points about inner critical voices and the tendency to revert to unhelpful behaviour patterns. A balance is necessary but examining the ways in which to build on strength is more positive than wallowing in memories of weakness. He argues that a move from 'fixing to flourishing' (Ghaye, 2010, p. 12) would be a novel and more constructive way of moving forward. This approach is conducive to building resilience, doing better in the workplace and promoting health. Therefore, application of these reflective ideas to your patients and service users and to yourself takes you forward and avoids a sticking point.

A number of reflective models or cycles have been utilised in healthcare education over the years. Gibbs (1988) has traditionally been popular in health and education. Gibbs (1988) asks that we first describe the incident and remember the associated feelings. Following an honest acknowledgement of feelings, we can examine the positives and negatives of the situation and then analyse how our actions affected communication and collaboration with the patient. A conclusion and action plan, based on knowledge about communication skills, identify how practice can be improved in the future.

Gibbs's reflective cycle

- Description: what happened?
- Feelings: how did you feel?
- Evaluation: weigh up the pros and cons.
- Analysis: what happened? Unpick what went on.
- Conclusion: what else could have been done?
- Action plan: what will you do next time?

Oelofson (2012) introduces another simple but effective model:

- Curiosity
- Looking closer
- Transformation.

Curiosity involves asking all the relevant questions about what happened within a situation. Looking closer invites the practitioner to reflect and consider alternative perspectives. Transformation means using the insights from the previous stages to embark on meaningful change. Oelofson (2012) stresses the importance of taking a reflective approach to practice. Students and qualified practitioners will find themselves in situations that will test their emotions as well as their skills. They are also required to facilitate positive change with service users. He argues that reflective practice helps nurses look after their own needs, whilst enhancing their capacities to work with service users.

Ghaye argues that reflective models must not only reflect but also enable change. Appreciative reflection and appreciative action, as outlined by Ghaye and Lillyman (2010, p. 11), have four tenets:

1. Appreciative intent towards knowing: focusing on our own and others' abilities
2. Appreciative intent towards relating: dialogue with others focused on a recognition of value and worth
3. Appreciative intent towards action: focusing on reaching the full potential of the individual, group or community
4. Appreciative intent towards organising: focusing on trust building and going forward in an emotionally intelligent manner, recognising that things may need to be done in different and innovative ways.

These involve awareness, i.e. reflecting not only on what is but also on how things could be; astuteness – interpretation and pragmatic implementation arising from awareness; and alignment – ensuring a match between what is said and what is done, and also alignment with the other person's, group's or community's need.

We recommend that you, as a student practitioner, should experiment with different reflective models to find the ones that work best for you. Reflective practice is an essential tool to help both improve communication and collaboration skills and to increase self-awareness and psychological wellbeing in a challenging but rewarding profession. Student story 2.2 is a comment from a student who reflected on how difficult life could be for patients with long-term conditions such as Chronic Obstructive Pulmonary Disease.

Student story 2.2: Life with a long-term condition

First, I noticed lots of negative reports on the care given in A&E. It appeared that most COPD patients go to A&E in the middle of the night and experience long waiting times and often have to wait until morning to see a doctor and be sent home.

This was what the positive reports said: people who were seen quickly with kindness and respect were happy with the care they had received. I therefore wish to be knowledgeable about the symptoms and stresses of long-term conditions and treat them as quickly as possible with kindness and respect for the pain and stress they are experiencing.

(www.studentopinion.org/, 2016)

Critical debate 2.1: Reflection on communication

Think back to a situation in practice where you communicated with a service user:
    What did you do? How did the service user react? How did you feel?
    Looking closer, what communication skills did you use? How were these designed to enhance collaboration and shared decision making? Was it good enough? How do you compare to other students/qualified staff?
    On reflection and with the new knowledge you have acquired, how might you transform your collaborative communication style next time?

 Visit the Values Exchange website at http://sagecomms.vxcommunity.com to develop your critical thinking skills and debate your thoughts and decisions.

Conclusion

In conclusion, this chapter has explored the building blocks of communication and showed that these require more focus and attention than might be commonly assumed. People may think that communication comes naturally but within a profession it requires particular forms. Professional identity and the need for repeated reflection on that identity have been highlighted. The benefits and also the potential dangers of 21st-century forms of electronic communication were examined. Social media have brought advantages in terms of easier communication but also potential dangers for students or professionals who do not take care to separate their social and professional profiles. This chapter finally looked at how students can begin to reflect on their own abilities with regard to communication, compassion and collaboration. Reflection is a subject to which we will return as it is one of the essential tools in the professional's repertoire to aid growth and development.

Further suggested activity

Explore resources on reflection. Try to find a model that works for you and practise reflecting on your own communicative practice. See, for example:

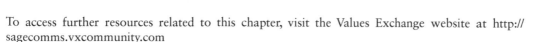

Journal of Reflective Practice: International and Multidisciplinary Perspectives
Flying Start NHS – www.flyingstart.scot.nhs.uk/
NICE on reflective practice – www.evidence.nhs.uk/search?q=reflective%20practice%20in%20nursing
Patient Opinion home page – www.patientopinion.org.uk/

To access further resources related to this chapter, visit the Values Exchange website at http://sagecomms.vxcommunity.com

References

Boud, D., Keogh, R. and Walker, D. (1985) *Turning Experience into Learning.* London: Kogan Paul.

Bulman, C. and Shutz, S. (2013) *Reflective Practice in Nursing.* Chichester: Wiley.

Chin, T. (2012) 'How nurses can use social media responsibly', *Nursing Times,* 108(29): 12–13.

Chomsky, N. (1979) *Language and Responsibility.* New York: Pantheon Books.

Clyne, W., Granby, T. and Picton, C. (2007) A *Competency Framework for Shared Decision Making with Patients: Achieving Concordance for Taking Medicines.* London: Medicines Partnership Programme at the National Prescribing Centre.

Cornford, T., Dean Franklin, B., Savage, I., Barber, N. and Jani, Y. (2009) *Electronic Prescribing in Hospitals: Challenges and Lessons Learned.* Available at: www.lse.ac.uk/LSEHealthAndSocialCare/pdf/information%20systems/eprescribing_report.pdf (accessed 17 April 2016).

Dougherty, L. and Lister, S. (2011) *The Royal Marsden Hospital Manual of Clinical Nursing Procedures,* 7th edn. Chichester: Wiley-Blackwell.

Gault, I. (2009) 'Service-user and carer perspectives on compliance and compulsory treatment in community mental health services', *Health and Social Care in the Community,* 17(5): 504–13.

Ghaye, A. (2010) *Teaching and Learning through Reflective Practice: A Practical Guide for Positive Practice.* London: Routledge.

Ghaye, A. and Lillyman, S. (2010) *Reflection: Principles and Practice for Healthcare Professionals.* London: Quay Books.

Gibbs, G. (1988) *Learning by Doing: A Guide to Teaching and Learning Methods.* London: Further Education Unit.

Ho, P.M., Bryson, C.L. and Rumsfeld J.L. (2009) 'Medication adherence: its importance in cardiovascular outcomes', *Circulation,* 119: 3028–35.

Johnson, M., Cowin, L., Wilson, I. and Young, H. (2012) 'Professional identity and nursing: contemporary theoretical developments and future research challenges', *International Nursing Review,* 59: 562–9.

Kozier, B., Erb, G., Berman, A., Snyder, S., Harvey, S. and Morgan-Samuel, H. (2012) *Fundamentals of Nursing: Concepts, Process and Practice,* 2nd edn. Harlow: Pearson Education.

Lambert, V. (2012) 'Theoretical foundations of communication', in V. Lambert, T. Long and D. Kelleher (eds), *Communication Skills for Children's Nurses.* Maidenhead: McGraw-Hill Education.

Mann, K., Gordon, J. and McLeod, A. (2009) 'Reflection and reflective practice in health professions education: a systematic review', *Advances in Health Science Education,* 14: 595–621.

McCabe, C. and Timmins, F. (2006) 'How nurse managers let down staff', *Nursing Management*, 13(3): 30–5.

McKewan, A. and Harris, G. (2010) *Communication Skills for Adult Nurses*. London: McGraw-Hill.

Montague, E., Chen, P.Y., Xu, J., Chewning, B. and Barrett, B. (2013) 'Nonverbal interpersonal interactions in clinical encounters and patient perceptions of empathy', *Journal of Participatory Medicine*, 5. Available at: www.jopm.org/evidence/research/2013/08/14/nonverbal-interpersonal-interactions-in-clinical-encounters-and-patient-perceptions-of-empathy/ (accessed 6 October 2015).

Nursing and Midwifery Council (NMC) (2015) *Guidance on Using Social Media Responsibly*. London: NMC.

Oelofson, N. (2012) 'Using reflective practice in frontline nursing', *Nursing Times*, 108(24): 22–4.

Okuda, R. and Fukada, M. (2014) 'Change resulting from reflective dialogues on nursing practice', *Yonago Actica Medica*, 57: 15–22.

Parliamentary and Health Service Ombudsman (2011) *Listening and Learning: The Ombudsman's Review of Complaint Handling by the NHS in England 2010–11*. Available at: www.ombudsman.org.uk/__data/assets/pdf_file/0019/12286/Listening-and-Learning-Screen.pdf (accessed 17 April 2016).

Quereshi, N., Al Dosssari, D., Al Zaagi, I., Al Bedah, A., Abdulli, A. and Koenig, H. (2015) 'Electronic health records, electronic prescribing and medication errors: a systematic review', *British Journal of Medical Research*, 5(5): 672–704.

Royal College of Nursing (2012) *Delegating Record Keeping and Countersigning Records: Nursing Guidelines*. London: RCN.

Schmidt Bunkers, S. (2010) 'The power and possibility in listening', *Nursing Science Quarterly*, 23(1): 22–7.

Schön, D. (1983) *The Reflective Practitioner*. New York: Basic Books.

Sikorski, W. (2012) 'Paralinguistic communication and the therapeutic relationship', *Archives of Psychiatry and Psychotherapy*, 1: 49–54.

Tolley, R. (2012) 'An overview of e-prescribing in secondary care', *Nursing Standard*, 26(22): 35–8.

Wren, C. (2012) 'An issue of confidence: social media for nurses and midwives', *The Guardian*, 21 February. Available at: www.theguardian.com/healthcare-network/2012/feb/21/issue-confidence-social-media-training (accessed 17 April 2016).

3

The Role of Attachment Theory and Cognition in Influencing Behaviour

Armin Luthi and Iris Gault

• • • • • • • • • • • • Learning Objectives • • • • • • • • • • • •

By the end of this chapter, you will have developed an understanding of:

- the role of cognition
- attachment theory
- understanding attachment, cognition and practice.

Don't forget to visit the Values Exchange website at http://sagecomms.vxcommunity.com for extra practice and revision activities.

• •

Introduction

A range of different theories and approaches has been developed by psychologists, counsellors and psychotherapists. This chapter focuses on developmental theories of cognition and attachment. These form the basis of a working theoretical template applicable in a wide range of clinical settings with a focus on beliefs and expectations. These theories provide understanding of the psychological and biological nuts and bolts of human thinking processes and the possibility of enabling people to develop more flexible and collaborative ways of managing and coping with illness and distress. Cognitive developmental theory and attachment theory enable exploration of our own and others' communicative interactions. Chapter 3 examines how thinking processes and early bonding experiences go on to influence our adult communication. The chapter will define and explore the role of cognition, focusing on Piaget, and then go on to outline Bowlby's attachment theory. Finally, it will examine cognition and attachment in relation to clinical practice.

The role of cognition

Student story 3.1: Gemma

Gemma is a student child field nurse. She's thrilled to have got a place on her course as there are not so many places for children's nursing and competition is fierce. She is in year 1 and enjoying the university part of the course so far. Gemma always knew she wanted to be a children's nurse as she loves babies and children. She entered nurse education straight after A levels. She did well at school and is considered to be quite academic so she feels reasonably confident that she can cope with the theoretical elements of the course. However, she is a bit more concerned with the prospect of practice. Although she thinks she will really enjoy interacting with the children, she realises there is more to nursing than that. She feels that she looks young (she is young at 19) and worries about looking and sounding authoritative enough. Will the parents of the children take her seriously? She is the youngest child in her own family and has always been the 'baby' of the family. Now, she will be expected to look after others and to sound like she knows what she's doing. Gemma keeps having thoughts such as 'I look like a schoolgirl', 'I wish I looked older', 'Can I really do this?' She is getting quite anxious at the thought of going out into practice.

 Visit the Values Exchange website at http://sagecomms.vxcommunity.com for a broader discussion on Gemma's story.

Cognition means thinking and reasoning. All human intellectual and brain activity is cognition (Sloman and Lagnado, 2015). Piaget (1977) developed cognitive theory in the 20th century and it remains a key area of study and practice in psychology. Piaget was extremely important in the development of cognitive theory. However, as is the case with theory, it is tested, disputed, refined and developed. Since his original observations of his own children in Austria in the early part of the 20th century, others have critiqued and evolved cognitive approaches.

Piaget studied the development of thinking or cognition in children and argued that schemas are the building blocks of knowledge and how we make sense of the world. These relate to everything we encounter and develop in numbers and sophistication as we develop and mature. Assimilation is the process by which new knowledge is taken in and understood. If existing schema cannot explain that new knowledge, the process of accommodation enables the schema to be changed to take in that new knowledge. Whilst our schema is managing to assimilate and accommodate knowledge, we are in a state of comfortable equilibrium, and we are in an uncomfortable state of disequilibrium when not managing to assimilate and accommodate. We therefore seek equilibrium in our mental processes of managing to explain the world.

Piaget advanced the theory that human cognition develops in distinct stages. Some argue that the stages are not entirely correct and that children develop more quickly. Others point out that his observations led him to generalise to all children in a manner that would not be accepted today (Slater and Bremner, 2011). It has been noted that not all adults progress through all stages. Vygotsky (1978) argued that the social and cultural factors must be taken into account. However, it is accepted that all theory and knowledge develop over time and that Piaget's work forms a valuable basis for our knowledge about cognition and the useful cognitive techniques we can use to improve healthcare communication (Slater and Bremner, 2011).

Piaget's cognitive stages

- **Sensory motor stage**: birth to 2 years – babies are largely reflexive and learn by responding to movements and manipulating objects. They are egocentric (concerned with themselves). In the early stages, they act as if an object no longer exists if it is hidden but develop the concept of object permanence as they mature.
- **Pre-operational stage**: 2–7 years – children expand their vocabulary and can take account of others. They remain egocentric but gradually realise they are not the centre of the universe. However, they believe that everyone else is like them.
- **Concrete operational stage**: 7–11 years – children begin to develop more logical thought. They can begin to appreciate that objects may not be the way they seem (conservation), that they can change, and they use their imagination to change scenarios. They become less egocentric (although this is not always the case with all).
- **Formal operational stage**: 11–16 years – these are the adolescent years when problem solving and propositional thought develop (they can consider the possibilities of an issue, even if a concrete object is absent; again, this may not be observed in all).

Cognitive therapies have become useful tools in addressing problematic thinking and communication within healthcare (Craske, 2010). Examples of health issues include areas where behaviour adversely affects health, such as overeating, risky alcohol consumption, failing to follow instructions or take prescribed medication. Our own communication and that of our patients is influenced by our thinking and reasoning processes. Thoughts can be helpful or unhelpful. It is important to understand that cognitive theory has several key messages to give us, and that these messages need to underline all of our therapeutic communications; the first one is especially important. Everyone who has a mind will, very often, find themselves having thoughts, ideas and beliefs that are strange, baffling and even disturbing. There is nothing wrong with this, as it just shows that our minds are working.

CRITICAL THINKING EXERCISE 3.1
RANDOM IDEAS

- Stop and check yourself, right now. What random ideas are floating through your mind?
- Identify these and write down at least a couple.

Second, our minds are constantly having these thoughts, ideas and beliefs because that is what our minds are designed to do. Minds are, by their very nature, creative and it is this creativity that has enabled us to survive so well as a species. Therefore, it is essential that we don't allow ourselves to become worried, scared or alienated by all these ideas and images – they are just demonstrating that our imaginations are working!

Third, our creativity is designed to help us identify and solve problems. These problems are often risky or dangerous in some way, due, of course, to the fact that life itself is intrinsically risky. Hence, nearly all the great innovations and inventions our minds have created for us have improved our survivability, solving issues of famine, illness and security in order to increase our lifespans and quality of life accordingly. In fact, it is useful to think of all of our thought processes as a problem-solving operation in one way or another. We are therefore completely indebted to our creativity as it has helped us to survive so well.

However, this great strength is also potentially a great weakness too. Things go wrong when we lose our ability to observe and analyse our thoughts and instead start to treat them as if they were real. By 'real', we mean cast in stone, and fixed, rigid and unchange-able. So, instead of reflecting on the many strange and often unhelpful things we say to ourselves, we start to act as though they are true, and this is where the trouble starts (Craske, 2010).

CRITICAL THINKING EXERCISE 3.2
SELF-CRITICAL THINKING – DOES THIS
HAPPEN TO YOU?

For instance, when we look in a mirror and see that we are looking tired, all kinds of ideas enter our minds. Instead of just being aware of being tired looking, we immediately start making all kinds of infer-ences, interpretations and judgements about looking tired. This then leads to us feel all kinds of strong emotions (anger, shame, sorrow, disgust, etc.) that have nothing to do with being tired looking, but are the result of our *beliefs* about being tired looking. And these are usually harsh and critical (e.g. 'it's bad to be tired looking', 'it's wrong to be tired looking', 'it's unattractive to be tired looking', 'other people don't like it if you are tired looking'). Have you noticed yourself do this? We are all, as they say, our own worst enemy, and this usually shows itself most clearly in the way we view ourselves in relation to other people, as we always put ourselves down, or compare ourselves unfavourably to others.

Self-critical thinking can be one of the key reasons that people struggle to care for them-selves and engage in unhelpful or self-defeating health behaviours such as consuming harmful substances (note that some recent research includes sugar in the list of such sub-stances; see Malhotra et al., 2015). This process occurs in patients and service users but often also in us – healthcare workers.

CRITICAL THINKING EXERCISE 3.3
DO YOU FEEL ABLE TO CHANGE
YOUR BEHAVIOUR?

Imagine for a minute that you wanted to try something new, something you had never tried before, and which you believed was beyond your abilities. What is likely to go through your mind? 'Oh yes, I'll have a go at that.'
   OR
   'Oh no, I can't do that'? Or 'If I even dare to try it then I will fail'? Or 'That's horrible! I don't want to even think about it'?
   How would you feel? And how likely is it that you would give it a go?

Many people find it difficult to have the faith or self-belief needed to make the required changes. In the next section, let's look at why this might be.

Attachment theory

Attachment theorists tell us that the roots of this self-criticism lie in our earliest experiences, when we were babies, so they focus on the impact our early bonding experiences have on our future self-esteem. Positive bonding with caregivers results in a positive self-image and effective communication patterns later in life. However, a poor bonding experience can negatively affect self-esteem and interactions with others. Our brains are divided into three sections: the hypothalamus (the reptile brain responsible for basic functions), the mid-brain (the primate brain responsible for basic relational functions) and the frontal brain (the human brain responsible for our higher human functions, e.g. morality). Only 25% of the frontal brain is formed at birth, and the rest develops as a direct consequence of nurturing. This area is seen to be the seat of our personalities, and so that nurturing experience makes a huge difference to adult functioning (Bowlby, 1983).

As babies, we all went through a learning process that helped us to become more autonomous and aware, both as a result of brain development and how we were cared for as our brains developed. Attachment theorists say that there is no such thing as a perfect nurturing experience (as otherwise no one would ever leave their parents!), but with 'good enough' nurturing resulting in secure attachment, a secure base is developed (Holmes, 2014).

Bowlby's (1969/1982) attachment theory sets out conditions that influence helpful or unhelpful attachment patterns. Our behaviour in later years is influenced by our experience of a parent's or parent substitute's actions.

Bowlby's attachment theory

If the child feels:

- positive and loved, this results in a secure attachment

or

- unloved and rejected, this results in an avoidant attachment

or

- angry and confused, this results in a resistant attachment.

What does having a secure base mean?

It is a working model of mind, by which, by being nurtured well, the infant builds the confidence to move towards taking control of their body (learning to walk, feed and toilet themselves), let other people know how they feel (through spoken communication) and come to understand that other people exist in the world apart from themself (and learn how to relate and empathise with them). This is all a very complex and difficult process, with lots of tears and tantrums on the way. A good enough carer is able to offer consistent, unconditional and secure nurturing in order to build esteem and confidence in the child during this time. Therefore, it represents nurturing that creates a sense of being loved or attached or bonded enough to other people so that we feel able to reach our full potential, so that we ensure that we utilise every opportunity given to us, and do not feel overly devastated when things don't work or go wrong. Bowlby's theories were influential in education and healthcare. As with Piaget, his work has been challenged and adapted. Some claim that his theories were used to suggest that women should not work when children are young in order not to risk the infant developing insecure attachments. However, Rutter (1981) and others have conducted research and refined the theory to demonstrate that, provided children have positive and consistent caregiving, it need not be the sole responsibility of the mother (Holmes, 2014).

Attachment theory has shown us that the nurturing experience we have is an essential part of our future personal identity or personality. When children do not have a good enough attachment/bonding experience, they tend to develop a mindset (or working model) about themselves, other people and the world that follows one of a number of patterns:

1. They become anxious and avoidant, tending to have very low confidence and unable to cope with stress and/or responsibility.
2. They become detached, tending to have very low confidence and so distancing themselves from stress and/or responsibility.
3. Or they become ambivalent, tending to have very low confidence and so getting themselves enraged and/or despairing in the face of stress and responsibility.

Whilst these patterns develop in childhood, they go on to become imprinted in the child's developing brain (as it goes through neuro-anatomical changes). The brain grows after birth, and because of its plasticity it never really stops growing. However, certain long-standing structural developments will remain consistent over time, especially in an area of the brain known as the limbic system.

Attachment and neuroanatomy: the limbic system

The limbic system is asserted to be the area of the brain responsible for our emotions and sociability/relationships. As with all theory and science, knowledge changes over time. There is some debate amongst scientists as to whether there is empirical evidence of a defined limbic system, as the anatomical structures are now seen differently to that of Broca in 1878 and Papez in 1937 (cited in Rajmohan and Mohandas, 2007). Nevertheless, as Rajmohan and Mohandas (2007) note, there is still much evidence that these parts of the brain are important for the study of emotion and control of emotion.

The limbic system

Its primary structures are:

- **the amygdala**: this regulates emotion, learning and memory and is key to the development of emotionally intuitive communication such as body language and facial expression.
- **the hippocampus**: this is essential for recall and memory, helping us to access and retrieve stored memories and knowledge. It is also very important in language development.
- **the hypothalamus**: this is the 'reptile brain' that regulates much of the autonomic/unconscious nervous system, and is responsible for our basic drives such as hunger, sexual arousal, blood pressure, heart rate, sleep, etc.

- **the middle prefrontal regions**: these regulate attention, awareness, self-regulation and the integration of thoughts and feelings.
- **the thalamus**: this regulates alertness and arousal.

The brain is an extremely complex 'system of systems' that is based on internal messaging and communication between the many structures and systems that together provide us with the functions that we generally summarise as the mind and body interface. This process only works because of a range of naturally produced chemical messengers that are constantly darting through our brains and bodies called neurotransmitters.

The brain is comprised of billions of nerve cells called neurons, and these share information and talk to each other through these chemical messengers. They help with the wiring of the brain connections and ensure that information is efficiently carried throughout the whole neural system. Again, how this system develops is strongly affected by the attachment experiences of the developing child, and several of these neurotransmitters are indelibly influenced by early life development.

Neurotransmitter messengers

These include:

- **Cortisol**: this is a stress messenger released by the adrenal gland. It leads to arousal and vigilance.
- **Dopamine**: this is a reward messenger that is essential in the processing of pleasant and rewarding sensations and experiences. It is a motivating chemical.
- **Serotonin**: this is an emotional messenger that plays a key role in mood/emotional regulation. It is a motivating chemical.
- **Norepinephrine**: this is an arousing messenger, designed to boost alertness and awareness.
- **Epinephrine or adrenaline**: the classic 'fight or flight' messenger, focusing attention and heightening fear responses.
- **Neuropeptides**: endorphins – the pain-killing messenger – are stress-reducing analgesic opioids that inure us to pain.
- **GABA** (gamma aminobutryc acid): the relaxing messenger that creates calm and sedation.
- **Oxytocin**: the attaching messenger that boosts nurturing, intimacy and care.
- **Vasopressin**: the relaxing messenger that increases bonding as well.

All of these neurotransmitters are highly sensitive to environmental cues such as sunlight (serotonin) or substances such as alcohol or cannabis (dopamine, serotonin, GABA), and due to their dynamic nature their levels are constantly changing. However, if a child is in a situation of constant stress, fear or neglect, then certain transmitters predominate – the stress transmitters – and it is believed that these then have a knock-on effect on how the overall limbic system then takes shape, leading to a system of systems that is over-exposed to messages of stress and negativity, which then shapes how the limbic system processes future perceptions, expectations and beliefs about the world. Therefore, a mixture of psychological, social and biological factors can mean that some reach adulthood with poor self-esteem and maladaptive communication and coping skills (Litwack, 2010).

Understanding attachment, cognition and practice

The theory explored above is helpful in understanding our own reactions and those of the service users and patients in our care. However, it is necessary to note that this is not simply dead theory and these issues are very much alive in contemporary practice. Researchers and clinicians are currently exploring how health (physical and mental) is linked to our cognitive and attachment styles, and are developing therapies.

The manner in which one thinks is perhaps unsurprisingly linked to the ability to succeed academically. Nozari and Siamian (2015) found that cognitive styles are closely related to academic success. Addressing thinking styles therefore may have a beneficial effect on children and young people. Early experience affects the capacity to function as a healthy adult and may have an impact on future mental and physical health. Roley et al. (2015) found that problematic thinking styles were closely related to post-traumatic stress disorder (PTSD) and depression.

Within physical healthcare, it has been found that psychological functioning has an impact on the ability to manage and cope with the diagnosis and management of symptoms. Shimizu et al. (2015) discovered links between cognitive coping skills and anxiety in lung cancer patients. Huang et al. (2016) found that cognitive coping styles were important in influencing how patients managed their type 2 diabetes. Regier and Parmelee's (2015) study on older people identified that cognitive traits had an effect on the ability to tolerate arthritic pain and the subsequent risk of developing depressive symptoms.

Much work is being conducted to examine how attachment affects adult experience. Pietromonaco et al. (2006) explore how infant bonding affects the ability to maintain adult relationships. Insecure attachments appear to result in difficulty with the regulation of emotions and can compromise future relationships. Davies et al. (2009) conducted a study to examine how early attachment experiences affected pain levels. This was a small-scale qualitative study but it found positive associations between perceptions of great pain and poor early bonding.

Obesity is becoming a significant problem for health services in the developed world. Taube-Schiff et al. (2015) found that patients undergoing bariatric surgery for weight-loss purposes tended to be emotional eaters. Their study found positive associations between poor early attachment, difficulty with emotional regulation and the development of unhealthy eating patterns as adults. Gerson et al. (2015) studied the characteristics of patients with irritable bowel syndrome, finding that attachment anxiety and avoidance scores were significantly higher than for those in the control group.

Costa-Martins et al. (2014) found that attachment styles were influential in the experience of pain during labour and consequently the need for pain relief. Ikeda et al. (2014) studied mothers' attachment styles and associations between this and the likelihood of developing postnatal depression. They found that problematic attachment was significantly linked to mood disorders. They suggest that screening for attachment style in pregnancy might help identify those most at risk.

A variety of psychological therapies have been developed to help those with psychological and physical distress (we shall be exploring these further in the book). Krahé et al. (2014) studied how certain forms of psychosocial support were helpful to patients with musculoskeletal pain and insecure attachments. Sandage et al. (2015) found that service users with borderline personality disorders could be helped to overcome the effects of insecure and anxious attachment with dialectical behaviour therapy.

Students at earlier stages of their programme will not be conducting research but are expected to begin to look at the literature in their subject areas. These studies indicate that there is considerable potential to improve health by understanding our cognitive and attachment styles.

In the meantime, there are some fairly simple measures that you can take within your own practice.

CRITICAL THINKING EXERCISE 3.4
THOUGHTS

Thoughts are just that – thoughts. They are not reality.

Thoughts are random and uncontrollable, and so attempting to alter, change or block them is an impossible and frustrating business.

Thoughts do matter as they are pivotal to how we see ourselves, other people and the world in general.

But our brains are designed to help us survive through problem solving, and so a lot of worrying thoughts are actually misplaced attempts at problem solving (but for problems that might not actually exist anywhere except in our minds).

We may create problems for ourselves by misconstruing events.

Our reasoning is frameworked by the schema or core beliefs and expectations that we develop in early childhood, and is based on our attachment experience from that time.

This means that our core beliefs and expectations are with us all our lives and the less helpful ones are likely to reappear when we are stressed (and naturally revert to more childlike thinking).

However, they can be moderated in a number of clear, systematic ways:

- Is it a fact, or just a thought?
- What am I actually reacting to?
- Is there another way of seeing this situation?
- How would someone I respect and admire think about that and react to that thought?
- What advice would I give to someone else in this situation?

We can learn to reduce unhelpful thinking habits, accept thoughts and so reduce their emotional impact.

CRITICAL THINKING EXERCISE 3.5
THOUGHTS, COGNITION AND ATTACHMENT

Self-critical thoughts only matter if we allow them to matter.

Thoughts can't be controlled, but they can be challenged.

We can challenge our thoughts in very simple ways.

Piaget showed how we develop our understanding ... lots of it is very ambiguous ... we like simple answers,

As Bowlby observed, a secure base allows us to be more flexible.

An insecure base may explain problematic behaviour.

Exploring this can help to regulate emotion.

Critical debate 3.1

Do nurses and midwives really need all this theory? Isn't this essentially a practical occupation?

What are the arguments for and against nurses and midwives learning and applying psychological theory?

Conclusion

In conclusion, psychological theory helps us understand thinking and how early emotional experience is helpful in enabling the nurse/midwife to know themselves and their coping styles. This is important so that we can anticipate and monitor our own communicative styles. Theories of cognition and of attachment are important in understanding our own and others' communicative interactions. These theories explain the psychobiological processes that affect all humans and point to where there may be problems. The effects of problematic cognition and attachment are evident in everyday clinical settings but can be ameliorated through a variety of psychological therapies and techniques. Troublesome thinking is simply troublesome thinking and does not have to become a reality. Understanding these processes is the first step in enabling more positive communication and behaviour.

Further suggested activity

How do you think about yourself? Explore psychological theory to determine: (1) how your thinking affects your behaviour; and (2) what type of attachment style you have. The following resources may help with this:

Cognitive Behaviour Therapy journal – www.tandfonline.com
NICE on psychological theory – www.evidence.nhs.uk/Search?q=psychological+theory
Royal College of Psychiatrists on CBT – www.rcpsych.ac.uk/mentalhealthinformation/therapies/cognitivebehaviouraltherapy.aspx
The Bowlby Centre (Psychotherapy Training and Referrals Organisation) home page – thebowlbycentre.org.uk

 To access further resources related to this chapter, visit the Values Exchange website at http://sagecomms.vxcommunity.com

References

Bowlby, J. (1969/1982) *Attachment and Loss, Vol. I*. New York: Basic Books.
Bowlby, J. (1983) *Attachment*. London: The Persus Book Group.
Costa-Martins, J.M., Pereira, M., Martins, H., Moura-Ramos, M., Coelho, R. and Tavares, J. (2014) 'The influence of women's attachment style on the chronobiology of labour pain, analgesic consumption and pharmacological effect', *Chronobiology International*, 31(6): 787–96.
Craske, M. (2010) *Cognitive Behavioural Therapy*. New York: American Psychological Therapy Association.
Davies, K., Macfarlane, G. and Dickens, C. (2009) 'Insecure attachment is associated with widespread, chronic pain', *Pain*, 143: 3–24.

Gerson, C., Gerson, M., Chang, L., Corazziari, E., Dumitrascu, D., Ghoshal, U., et al. (2015) 'A cross-cultural investigation of attachment style, catastrophising, negative pain beliefs, and symptom severity in irritable bowel syndrome', *Neurogastroenterology and Motility*, 27(4): 490–500.

Holmes, J. (2014) *The Search for the Secure Base: Attachment Theory and Psychotherapy*. London: Routledge.

Huang, C., Lai, H., Lu, Y., Chen, W., Chi, S., Lu, C. and Chen, C. (2016) 'Risk factors and coping style affect health outcomes in adults with Type 2 Diabetes', *Biological Research for Nursing*, 18: 82–9.

Ikeda, M., Hayashi, M. and Kamibeppu, K. (2014) 'The relationship between attachment style and postpartum depression', *Attachment and Human Development*, 16(6): 557–72.

Krahé, C., Paloyelis, Y., Sambo, C. and Fotopoulou, A. (2014) 'I like it when my partner holds my hand: development of the Responses and Attitudes to Support during Pain questionnaire (RASP)', *Frontiers of Psychology*, 5: 1027.

Litwack, G. (2010) *Hormones of the Limbic System*. San Diego, CA: Academic Press.

Malhotra, A., Noakes, T. and Phinney, S. (2015) 'It is time to bust the myth of physical inactivity and obesity: you cannot outrun a bad diet', *British Journal of Sports Medicine*, 49: 967–8.

Nozari, A. and Siamian, H. (2015) 'The relationship between field dependent–independent cognitive style and understanding of English text reading and academic success', *Materia Sociomedica*, 27(1): 39–41.

Piaget, J. (1977) *The Development of Thought*. New York: Viking Press.

Pietromonaco, P., Feldman, L. and Powers, S. (2006) 'Adult attachment theory and affective reactivity and regulation', in D. Snyder, J. Simpson and J. Hughes (eds), *Emotion Regulation in Couples and Families: Pathways to Dysfunction and Health*, pp. 57–74. Washington, DC: American Psychological Association.

Rajmohan, V. and Mohandas, E. (2007) 'The limbic system', *Journal of Psychiatry*, 49(2): 132–9.

Regier, N. and Parmelee, P. (2015) 'The stability of coping strategies in older adults with osteoarthritis and the ability of these strategies to predict changes in depression, disability, and pain', *Aging and Mental Health*, 6: 1–10.

Roley, M., Claycomb, M., Contractor, A., Dranger, P., Armour, C. and Elhai, J. (2015) 'The relationship between rumination, PTSD, and depression symptoms', *Journal of Affective Disorders*, 9(180): 116–21.

Rutter, M. (1981) *Maternal Deprivation Reassessed*, 2nd edn. London: Penguin Books.

Sandage, S., Long, B., Moen, R., Jankowski, P., Worthington, E., Wade, N. and Rye, M. (2015) 'Forgiveness in the treatment of borderline personality disorder: a quasi-experimental study', *Journal of Clinical Psychology*, 71: 625–40.

Shimizu, K., Nakaya, N., Saito-Nakaya, K., Akechi, T., Ogawa, A., Fujisawa. D., et al. (2015) 'Personality traits and coping styles explain anxiety in lung cancer patients to a greater extent than other factors', *Japanese Journal of Clinical Oncology*, 45(5): 456–63.

Slater, A. and Bremner, G. (2011) *An Introduction to Developmental Psychology*. Chichester: John Wiley & Sons.

Sloman, S. and Lagnado, A. (2015) 'Causality in thought', *Annual Review of Psychology*, 66(3): 1–3.

Taube-Schiff, M., Van Exan, J., Tanaka, R., Wnuk, S., Hawa, R. and Sockalingam, S. (2015) 'Attachment style and emotional eating in bariatric surgery candidates: the mediating role of difficulties in emotion regulation', *Eating Behaviours*, 28(18): 36–40.

Vygotsky, L. (1978) *Mind in Society*. Cambridge, MA: Harvard University Press.

4

Enabling Positive Health Behaviour

Armin Luthi and Iris Gault

• • • • • • • • • • • • • Learning Objectives • • • • • • • • • • • •

By the end of this chapter, you will have gained an introductory knowledge of:

* changing patterns of ill health and the need for successful health education communication
* motivational interviewing and its potential for collaborative behaviour change
* the role of emotional intelligence and mindfulness.

Don't forget to visit the Values Exchange website at http://sagecomms.vxcommunity.com for extra practice and revision activities.

• •

Introduction

This chapter explores some contemporary concerns in healthcare today and the need to practise more effectively. This involves treating patients and ourselves in kinder and more collaborative ways. Much ill health today is now associated with unhealthy behaviour. Despite acknowledgement that health promotion or education is an essential part of healthcare, conditions that could be ameliorated by behaviour change have proven resistant to intervention. Therefore, this chapter explores health education approaches focusing on motivational interviewing's role in understanding behaviour change. It will then invite the reader to reflect on their own wellbeing, suggesting that emotional intelligence and mindfulness are helpful as supportive strategies.

Student story 4.1: Molly

Molly is a student midwife in the first year of her course. She is enjoying the combination of theory and practice. Molly always knew she wanted to be a midwife as she loves babies

---

and likes the idea of working with mainly 'well' women rather than ill people. She came into midwifery straight from school. She got good grades at school and is getting on well with the academic work and the practice so far. However, she is a bit concerned about her next practice placement. Molly comes from a very middle-class background. Her mother is an academic and her father is a doctor and her world until now has been largely confined to people just like herself. Her next placement will be in the community in an area that is socially and economically deprived. She realises that she will be dealing with a number of very young parents-to-be. Part of the placement is with the specialist midwives who work with pregnant teenagers. This should be really interesting but the girls will be very different from the mainly 'yummy mummies' in the affluent area in her last in-patient placement. She will need to know all the theory but also how to communicate in a non-patronising manner. Health promotion is such an important part of antenatal care. Will she be taken seriously? Can she empathise with this group? Molly is thinking that she won't be able to do this very well and it is denting her confidence.

Changing patterns of ill health and health education

Health education can take many forms and the term 'health education' is often used interchangeably with 'health promotion'. We will persist with the term 'health education' as defined by the World Health Organization as 'any combination of learning experiences, designed to help individuals and communities improve their health, by increasing their knowledge or influencing their attitudes' (www.who.int/topics/health_education/en/, 2015). This acknowledges that there are very many useful techniques and that different situations will require different approaches.

There is a need for more effective health education in most countries but a particular need in the developed world where ill health is often related to our behaviour. The UK Department of Health (2012) examined the position regarding people with long-term conditions (LTCs) and concluded that the healthcare approaches taken had largely been ineffective to date. Examples of conditions that can be helped by health educational approaches include hypertension, diabetes, asthma, coronary heart disease, arthritis and most mental health conditions. It is also important to note that, in most cases, people with long-term conditions will have more than one condition, often a combination of physical and mental. Obesity is a factor in some of these conditions and affects all age groups. Maternal obesity is of concern, with approximately 50% of women of childbearing age officially classified as overweight or obese (www.noo.org.uk/NOO_about_obesity accessed 16 February 2016). It is, however, important not to victim-blame but to appreciate that many health problems can be alleviated or even prevented by behaviours such as diet control and/or emotional regulation.

These patients and service users with LTCs form 30% of the population but take up 70% of the budget, with 50% of all GP appointments and 64% of outpatient appointments (Department of Health, 2012). In addition, many of the same people have been reported to be those taken to Accident and Emergency (A&E) departments with exacerbations of their long-term condition that could or should have been managed in a community setting (Department of Health, 2012). Reasons for this state of affairs are varied and complex but there is consensus that our attempts to enable people to change and manage their own health behaviour have been limited in effect.

Coulter et al. (2013) explain that health services have traditionally had a reactive response to long-term health problems, focusing on acute episodes. This approach, however, tends to neglect people following the acute episode of care rather than exploring how the condition can be changed. Hibbard and Greene (2013) argue that there is much evidence to show that when people are enabled to become adept at understanding and managing their condition, there are positive results. This involves good education and support from professionals.

Coulter et al. (2013, p. 4) point out that professionals working in healthcare need to have skills that help patients to become knowledgeable about their condition and make collaborative decisions about care. They need to be able to offer the 'emotional, psychological and practical support' that moves the situation forward. This involves neither telling people to address their health behaviour such as sticking to a diet nor simply supplying sympathetic support. History demonstrates that advice and sympathy have produced poor results. The numbers of people living with long-term conditions that could be improved by behavioural change have increased to 15 million. This is not simply a matter for those dealing with older people. Although a growing ageing population has contributed to these numbers, the biggest figures are in those under 65 (Coulter et al., 2013). In Scotland, 42% of the population had one long-term condition and 23% were living with more than one (Barnett et al., 2012).

The roots of long-term conditions lie in childhood or even pre-conception. The behaviour of parents and parents-to-be influences the health of their children and there is evidence that this varies hugely between different areas and different social groups. In affluent parts of London (Westminster) smoking at the time of delivery has fallen to 2.1%, but has risen in more northerly parts of the country such as Blackpool where it is 26.2% (www.hscic.gov.uk/datacollections/ssatod). Compelling evidence from the Kings Fund suggests that these problems are getting worse (Buck and Mcguire, 2015). Therefore, there is little doubt that nurses and midwives require psychological understanding and very effective and focused communication skills to facilitate prospective parents and people with LTCs to improve their health. National Voices (2013) (a voluntary group representing patients) and Diabetes UK (2011) (similarly representing people with diabetes) have made clear that patients in these situations are keen to see a more patient-centred and collaborative care experience. National Voices (2013) has developed a 'gold standard' view of care that stresses the patient perspective should be the driving force behind all care decisions.

CRITICAL THINKING EXERCISE 4.1
COLLABORATIVE DECISION MAKING

How prepared are you to engage in collaborative decision making with a service user with problematic eating behaviour or chronic smoking that is adversely affecting their health? What skills might you require?

stages that have a circular pattern to them, and as a sort of carousel that we can step on or off at any time (and in fact do frequently).

Stages of change

- **Stage 1: pre-contemplation** – at this time we do not think that there is any need for change
- **Stage 2: contemplation** – we have started to consider making a change
- **Stage 3: preparation** – we have decided to make a change and prepare to do so
- **Stage 4: action** – we make the change
- **Stage 5: maintenance** – we sustain the change
- **Stage 6: relapse** – we no longer sustain the change, which takes us back to
- **Stage 1: pre-contemplation** – and so the cycle can begin (or not) again. (Prochaska and DiClemente, 1983, cited in Mason, 2005)

This approach is interested in what the person thinks and feels about change, but measures it in actual behaviour. This is a very important principle, because it helps us to appreciate that people will often spend a lot of time at the pre-contemplative stage, and then rapidly go through a cycle of change, because they have as yet not fully explored their ambivalence.

Let's demonstrate this with an example that is likely to apply to you.

CRITICAL THINKING EXERCISE 4.3
MOTIVATIONAL INTERVIEWING QUESTIONS (B)

Let's suppose it's 6.30 a.m. on a Monday morning and your alarm goes off, telling you that you have to be in nursing class at 09.00. As you slowly wake up, which stage are you at?

I bet its **PRE-CONTEMPLATION**, as you say to yourself, 'I don't want to get up, as I'm tired, and it's raining outside and the train will be packed, and it's a lecture on a boring subject, given by a boring lecturer', etc.

However, as you lie there, ambivalence develops. You remember that it is important for you to attend all your lectures as you are keen to develop your knowledge, and that it might be a boring subject to you, but it is also a core part of the curriculum.

This generates **CONTEMPLATION** and, as a result, you slowly get yourself out of bed and, as you **PREPARE** to get to class, you move into **ACTION** as you go out the door. Once at university, you are in **MAINTENANCE**. You get home, and later on, as you get tired, you go to bed. In the morning, at 6.30, your alarm goes off … you may **RELAPSE** and wake up in **PRE-CONTEMPLATION** again, and so the cycle starts all over again …

Visit the Values Exchange website at http://sagecomms.vxcommunity.com to develop your critical thinking skills and debate your thoughts and decisions.

Obviously, some people might feel differently about going to class and leap joyously out of bed at the chance, but we think you can still understand the situation and relate to it. The important thing to remember here is the ambivalence. Without being able to analyse and appraise the situation realistically, and weigh up the pros and cons, there is a risk that we'd all still be in bed!

This is a very important point to remember with your clients when undertaking health promotion. Always invite them to explore their ambivalence by carrying out a cost-benefit analysis of the situation, and encourage them to openly appraise their thoughts and feelings about their behaviours. Let's use our 'get out of bed' example again.

CRITICAL THINKING EXERCISE 4.4
MOTIVATION INTERVIEWING QUESTIONS (C)

What are the good things about staying in bed and phoning in sick to university?

I can sleep for longer. I can watch TV all day. I won't have to go out in the rain. I won't have to commute. I could catch up with my assignment, etc.

What are the bad things about staying in bed and phoning in sick to university?

I won't be able to go back to sleep now. I will miss the lectures. I might fall behind. I will miss a chance to see my colleagues. I will still have to go out in the rain because I need to do some shopping. I will get bored of TV after an hour or so. I will start to feel guilty after a while, etc.

If applied to our patients and service users, by using this cost-benefit analysis we are able to discuss their ambivalence without judgement, and enable them to consider their options from as wide a perspective as possible.

The role of emotional intelligence and mindfulness

Nursing and midwifery are challenging professions. A reason for the emphasis on compassionate and collaborative communication is the observation that both were found to be lacking in cases of poor care such as Mid staffordshire (Francis, 2013). However, in many instances of poor care, it is found that staff lack support and have low morale. This is no excuse but it is necessary to appreciate that in order to be kind to others, we need to first be kind to ourselves. Burnout is a danger where healthcare professionals do not attend to their own psychological wellbeing. Burnout was defined in Chapter 1 as a type of emotional blunting, resulting in an uncaring attitude (Zhang et al., 2014). Two areas of psychology are proving increasingly useful in nursing and midwifery communication: emotional intelligence and mindfulness.

Emotional intelligence and competence

First, we focus on emotional intelligence. Nursing is a discipline that we need to use skilfully, compassionately and intelligently, and to do this we need to apply compassion and intelligence to ourselves, before we can apply these to others. The concept of emotional intelligence was developed by Goleman (1996, cited in Riggio and Reichard, 2008) and is the term used to describe our ability to relate successfully to others. It is a complex process involving self-awareness, empathy, honesty and congruence. Its basics are learned when we are young, but we go on learning them throughout life. It is not, as Goleman (1999) says, about being 'nice'. Emotional intelligence requires us to be aware, mindful and in control of our emotions, so that we can remain empathically attuned to others. Essentially, having good emotional intelligence means that we are able to understand ourselves sufficiently well enough to understand others (no matter the circumstances). As a nurse, it is absolutely vital that you have good emotional intelligence. The nature of nursing means that we are mainly working with people/clients who are in emotional distress. Sometimes it might be that people are in tremendous physical pain. Sometimes it may be emotional pain. Sometimes the intensity of their pain might leave us feeling helpless and in pain ourselves, possibly because it reminds us of experiences from our own lives, or because we don't know what to say or do, or for any of a multitude of other reasons, and it is at those times that we cease to be competent practitioners. Let's think about this with another reflective exercise.

CRITICAL THINKING EXERCISE 4.5
EMOTIONAL INTELLIGENCE

How do you respond to people in pain? Why do you respond that way? And what led you to choose to respond in that way? And how effective is it?

Think about these questions for 10 minutes, writing down your reflections.

Emotional intelligence is complemented by emotional competence. Brasseur et al. (2013, p. 1) explain that emotional competence 'refers to how an individual identifies, expresses, understands, regulates and uses his emotions or those of others'. Goleman (1999) argues that it is possible to learn emotional competence, and that in some cases (or professions) it is unavoidable, due to the very nature of the work those professionals do. This means we must be fully aware of ourselves, in terms of our own personal attitudes, feelings, beliefs and values (about ourselves, other people and the world in general), and how these might influence and affect our professional attitudes, feelings, beliefs and values, because they are not automatically the same. Without this awareness, all of us can have emotional blind spots that can have profound repercussions, both for us and for those people we care about. So let's put this into practice with more reflective exercises.

CRITICAL THINKING EXERCISE 4.6
KNOWING YOURSELF

Do you feel that you truly know yourself? Can you guarantee, on a day-to-day basis, what your mood, expectations and attitude will be when you first wake up in the morning? Or are there lots of other things (what we call 'variables') that also decide this? Do you ever find yourself having strange or surprising ideas? Do you ever find yourself getting into an internal conflict about decisions you need to make?

(Continued)

(Continued)

Spend 10 minutes writing down your reflections (i.e. thoughts, memories and recollections).

On a scale of 1–10, rate your emotional intelligence and competence. Do you know yourself well enough to be aware of how your attitudes affect your interaction with others?

CRITICAL THINKING EXERCISE 4.7
EMOTIONAL COMPETENCE

Think back to your own experiences of receiving healthcare. How were you treated? Did you find that you were expected to be passive, compliant and obedient? How much time was given for you to ask questions? Or check on the details of what was being done? How did you feel about the overall experience?

Spend 10 minutes writing down your reflections.

Rate the practitioner on a scale of 1–10 on their emotional competence. How attentive were they to your needs?

Mindfulness

Next, we explore mindfulness as a means of both knowing ourselves and being kind to ourselves. Mindfulness is considered a useful tool in many areas of life including healthcare and education. Peña-Sarrionandia et al. (2015, p. 4) define it as 'purposefully paying attention to the present moment in a non-judgemental way. It consists in observing what is happening moment by moment in one's internal (thoughts, motives, emotions, bodily sensations) and external world, without judging it'. It originates from the spiritual world, most specifically Buddhism, but has been researched extensively and is gaining acceptance as a valid measure of improving psychological functioning (Killingworth and Gilbert, 2010). Therefore, mindfulness is the process by which we pay attention to our thoughts, feelings and bodies, and notice how it is affecting us. In essence, it is the means by which we understand what we are telling ourselves. However, to be effective, it is important to focus not only on what we feel (internal attention) but also on what we do (external attention) (Peña-Sarrionandia et al., 2015).

That could sound easy, and you are probably telling yourself right now that you already do it anyway, and of course you do. However, research shows us that stress, anxiety, fatigue and preoccupation mean that most of us, in fact, do not pay proper attention to ourselves at all. To start off this process, we can frame it simply by dividing our minds into three parts: the emotional mind; the logical mind; and the wise mind.

Minds

- **Emotional mind**: the sub-cortical more primitive brain. When this predominates, we tend to be hot-headed and ruled by emotions (and are likely to be emotionally over-involved).
- **Logical mind**: the frontal cortex that provides the logical, problem-solving function of the brain. When this predominates, we tend to be too cold and logical, dominated by thoughts (and are likely to be emotionally detached).

- **Wise mind**: the integration of the other two mindsets in order to strike the best, most compassionate balance (which is when we are acting with professional care). (Kabat-Zinn, 2013)

By using mindfulness, we can stay in the present and enjoy life for what it is, rather than allowing our emotional minds to take over. Too often, we overly focus on thinking of ideal scenarios in which everything will be perfect when we should be accepting the present situation. Mindfulness suggests that by doing this we will make better decisions. Kabat-Zinn (2013) writes:

> Like subterranean water, or vast oil deposits, or minerals buried deep within the rock of the planet, we are talking here of interior resources deep within ourselves, innate to us as human beings, resources that can be tapped and utilised, brought to the fore – such as our life long capacities for learning, for growing, for healing, and for transforming ourselves. And how might such a transformation come about? It comes directly out of our ability to take a larger perspective, to realise that we are bigger than who we think we are. It comes directly out of recognising and inhabiting the full dimensionality of our being, of being who and what we actually are. (2013, p. xxvi)

CRITICAL THINKING EXERCISE 4.8
MINDFULNESS

First, use your observing eye to ascertain how you are reacting to college, work and personal demands:

Emotional mind: are you using the emotional mind? Becoming overly and frantically focused on finishing the admin task, no matter how much it impacts on your client contact? And so a hamster in a wheel (in a state of heightened emotional mind)? Not stopping to think about the clinical implications of your actions?

Rational mind: or are you using the rational mind? Becoming a technician that needs to ignore clients in order to focus on the administrative and paperwork? No matter how much that then compromises client care?

Wise mind: we are problem solvers by nature and design. By using our observing eye, we engage the wise mind. This helps us analyse problems in order to solve them:

- What am I feeling?
- What are my priorities and how are my feelings impacting on my priorities?
- What is my number one priority?
- What is the worst possible outcome?
- How can I prevent the worst possible outcome?
- Which tasks are most important in preventing the worst outcome?

Accept that you are not superhuman; the situation may not be ideal but it can be reappraised in terms of what must be done now and what can be left till later.

Therefore, mindfulness is about accessing your full potential, discovering who you really are, and accepting who you really are, without judgement and with kindness. And we do it in the most simple way imaginable: we pause, take a breath and allow our mind to flow, without interrupting, censoring or stopping this. Instead, through mindfulness practice, we can learn to observe and understand, rather than judge, ourselves. Following on from this, we can then apply the same non-judgemental acceptance to service users and patients. This is important, as lacking self-awareness, not being mindful and being judgemental can be incredibly hurtful, as Patient story 4.1 indicates.

Patient story 4.1: 'Just because I'm young'

I had given birth to my daughter as a first time anxious mum. Ward staff were great until I moved to ward 7 and had the upset of meeting a member of staff who was horrible to me and made my life hell when I had given birth. When I first moved wards I asked the member of staff if they could help to feed my daughter, as I was not sure I was doing it properly. The member of staff said no and that I may as well learn for myself and walked away. The member of staff then commented some time later that younger women shouldn't be allowed to have kids to which I cried. Then my family had brought me flowers and chocolate when they visited which I was eating when the member of staff asked how much I weighed and could see I was overweight, to which I said it was nothing to do with them. The member of staff then said I shouldn't eat the chocolate, I was already big and hopefully my child wouldn't turn out big like me, and walked away laughing saying 'poor baby' a few times. Totally ruined the experience of it for me and the member of staff made me doubt myself as a mum and a human being. Will never give birth at ***** ******* again, amazing how one person's horrible treatment of me can ruin the whole experience just because I'm young.

(www.patientopinion.org.uk/, 2016)

Critical debate 4.1: Judging or not judging?

Is mindfulness just woolly-minded nonsense? Why do we need to know ourselves? Do you understand why the young mother was judged? OR was this unacceptable and, if so, what should happen next?

Remember that all patientopinion.org/ feedback is communicated to the relevant hospital trust in real time. How should a service respond to feedback about staff attitudes towards service users and patients?

Conclusion

In conclusion, this chapter has explored the changing requirements for contemporary healthcare. It has considered the increasing numbers of people living with poorly managed long-term conditions and the need for healthcare staff to develop more skilled and collaborative communication to facilitate a positive health behaviour change. Motivational interviewing – an approach that can be delivered in brief interventions as part of normal clinical practice – was outlined and applied. Finally, the chapter explored strategies for students and healthcare practitioners to help them not only improve practice but also to reach and maintain their own psychological wellbeing. In order to be communicatively kind to others, we must first be kind to ourselves.

Further suggested activity

Try practising mindfulness to see how it feels. To help you, explore the following resources:

Mindfulness journal – www.springer.com/psychology/cognitive+psychology/journal/12671?token= prtst0416p
Daniel Goleman on emotional intelligence – www.danielgoleman.info/topics/emotional-intelligence/
Oxford Mindfulness Centre – www.oxfordmindfulness.org
Psychology Today on emotional intelligence – www.psychologytoday.com/basics/emotional-intelligence
Visual maps showing how obesity has changed between 1996 and 2012 – www.noo.org.uk/visualisation/adult_obesity

To access further resources related to this chapter, visit the Values Exchange website at http://sagecomms.vxcommunity.com

References

Barnett, K., Mercer, S.W., Norbury, M., Watt, G., Wyke S. and Guthrie, B. (2012) 'Epidemiology of multimorbidity and implications for healthcare research and medical education: a cross sectional study', *The Lancet*, 380(3896): 37–43.

Brasseur, S., Gregoire, J., Boudu, R. and Mikolajzak, M. (2013) 'The profile of emotional competence: development and validation of a self-reported measure that fits dimensions of emotional competence theory', PLOS, 6 May. Available at: http://journals.plos.org/plosone/article?id=10.1371/journal.pone.0062635 (accessed 14 April 2016).

Buck, D and McGuire, D. (2015) *Inequalities in Life Expectancy: Changes Over Time and Implications for Policy*. London: The Kings Fund.

Coulter, A. Roberts, S. and Dixon, A. (2013) *Delivering Better Services for People with Long-term Conditions*. London: The Kings Fund.

Department of Health (DoH) (2012) *Long-term Conditions: Compendium of Information*. London: The Stationery Office.

Diabetes UK (2011) *Thanks for the Petunias: A Guide to Developing and Commissioning Non-traditional Providers to Support the Self-management of People with Diabetes*. London: Diabetes UK.

Francis, R. (2013) *Report of the Mid Staffordshire NHS Foundation Trust Public Inquiry*. London: The Stationery Office.

Goleman, D. (1999) *Working with Emotional Intelligence*. London: Bloomsbury.

Hibbard, J.H. and Greene, J. (2013) 'What the evidence shows about patient activation: better health outcomes and care experience; fewer data on costs', *Health Affairs*, 32(2): 207–14.

Kabat-Zinn, J. (2013) *Full Catastrophe Living*. New York: United Buddhist Church Inc.

Killingworth, S. and Gilbert, D. (2010) 'A wandering mind is an unhappy mind', *Science*, 330: 932–3.

Lundahl, B. and Burke, B. (2009) 'The effectiveness and applicability of motivational interviewing: a practice friendly review of four meta analyses', *Journal of Clinical Psychology*, 65(11): 1232–45.

Lundahl, B., Moleni, T., Burke, B., Butters, R., Tollefson, D., Butler, C. and Rollnick, S. (2014) 'Motivational interviewing in medical care settings: a systematic review and meta-analysis of randomized controlled trials', *University of York Centre for Dissemination and Review*. York: National Institute for Health Research.

Mason, P. (2005) 'Helping individuals change behaviour', in L. Ewles (ed.), *Key Topics in Public Health*. London: Churchill Livingstone. pp. 261–76.

Millar, W.R. and Rollnick, S. (2002) *Motivational Interviewing: Preparing People for Change*, 2nd edn. New York: Guildford Press.

National Voices (2013) *A Narrative for Person Centred Co-ordinated Care*. London: National Voices (www.noo.org.uk).

Nursing and Midwifery Council (NMC) (2010) *Standards for Professional Practice Pre-Registration*. London: NMC.

Peña-Sarrionandia, A., Mikolajczak, M. and Gross, J.J. (2015) 'Integrating emotional regulation and emotional intelligence traditions: a meta-analysis', *Frontiers in Psychology*, 6(160).

Riggio, R. and Reichard, R. (2008) 'The social and emotional intelligence of leadership', *Journal of Managerial Psychology*, 23(2): 169–85.

Zhang, X., Huang, D. and Guan, P. (2014) 'Job burnout among critical care nurses from 14 adult intensive care units in northeastern China: a cross-sectional survey', *British Medical Journal: BMJ Open*, 4(6): e004813.

Useful websites

Health & Social Care Information Centre (hscic) – www.hscic.gov.uk/World Health Organization on health education – www.who.int/topics/health_education/en/

CONCLUSION TO
PART 1

Part 1 examined the centrality yet complexity of communication in collaborative relationships with patients and service users. It considered how communication knowledge and skill are taken for granted until one is confronted by a patient in difficult circumstances. Similarly, the ability to co-operate and collaborate was shown to be much more demanding than commonly supposed. Chapter 2 went on to unpick the nuts and bolts of communication in order to start to demonstrate how these can be learned and practised effectively, provided the health professional also develops self-awareness. The components of professional communication in nursing and midwifery and the need for reflective practice have been outlined. The importance of beginning to distinguish between a professional and a social identity was highlighted. Part 1 then considered the role of developmental psychological theory in examining and explaining the processes that affect adult behaviour and communication patterns. In particular, emphasis was put on the role of cognition and attachment theory as important in explaining our own and others' behaviours. Contemporary health issues and the need to develop more effective forms of health behaviour change methods were examined; this is one of the most challenging issues facing healthcare services, yet relatively easy changes in professional communication could facilitate real change. Part 1 then concluded with one of the most important points: acknowledging and examining how it is essential that nurses and midwives look after their own psychological wellbeing, to avoid burnout and provide compassionate care for patients. Developing emotional intelligence and competence is an essential element of self-awareness, and using these and a mindful approach to looking after ourselves will enable more effective care and communication for patients and service users in the longer term.

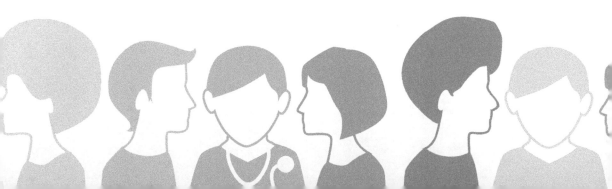

PART 2

COMMUNICATION SKILLS IN PRACTICE

Whereas Part 1 focused on you – the student nurse or midwife – Part 2 concentrates on the patient/service user or care group. This section does provide a variety of techniques and tools to address particular health issues, but in the main, we want students to understand that their communicative responses should be compassionate and context-specific. An appreciation of and empathy for the position of the patient/service user are what should underpin interaction. Although psychological tools are helpful in supplying a template for the health professional unsure of how to proceed, there is no substitute for knowledge, understanding and a genuine readiness to listen.

The context around each care group is discussed to highlight their specific needs. A major issue that influences communication with others is any stigma or stereotyping applied to that group. Stigmatising behaviour exists within society and, sadly, is often associated with illness and health behaviour. Therefore, where appropriate, the impact of stigma, both on the group and on professional communication, will be examined and challenged.

Part 2 begins with Chapter 5 on some of the common, yet crucial concerns in healthcare: examining how to address communication issues in acute and/or traumatising conditions and also exploring transformative approaches to health behaviour in long-term conditions. Chapter 6 looks at an area of healthcare arguably most vulnerable to stigmatising communication – that of mental health – and examines how to communicate in a non-discriminatory manner. Chapter 7 continues with that theme, exploring communication challenges for groups with cognitive deficits such as dementia, learning disability and head injury. The focus then switches to the lifespan and Chapter 8 concentrates on communication with families, children and young people. Chapter 9 continues with understanding the communication challenges of the middle-aged and older adult. (We have deliberately not included dementia in this chapter as it is not seen as an inevitable consequence of age.) Finally, Chapter 10 investigates one of the most sensitive areas of healthcare – that of palliative care and the provision of effective and supportive communication in very complex cases, including those in the terminal stages of life.

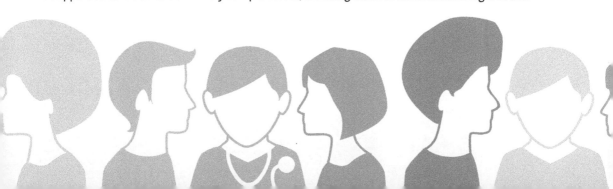

5

Communicating to Help Health Service Users Understand and Deal with their Condition

Iris Gault

• • • • • • • • • • • • Learning Objectives • • • • • • • • • • • •

By the end of this chapter, you will have developed have an understanding of:

- the importance of psychosocial care in contemporary health challenges
- communicating with patients who are anxious and/or distressed
- communicating with service users with long-term conditions to help change health behaviour.

Don't forget to visit the Values Exchange website at http://sagecomms.vxcommunity.com for extra practice and revision activities.

• •

Introduction

This chapter examines communication issues in common, yet pressing conditions in contemporary healthcare. There are two main sections, with the first half of this chapter devoted to issues around helping patients deal with psychological distress when faced with challenging, acute and life-threatening health conditions. Nurses often feel worried about how to respond to those facing such conditions and some patients report poor psychological care (Legg, 2011). Examples of training in psychosocial support taken from acute and secondary care, mainly in cancer services, demonstrate how nurses and midwives can adapt their communication to provide helpful emotional assistance.

The second part of the chapter goes on to consider an equally challenging issue – how to positively deal with patients and service users with long-term conditions. As reported in Part 1, these patients comprise 30% of the healthcare population but take up 70% of the budget (House of Commons Health Committee, 2014). They can become stuck in a cycle of behaviour that exacerbates their health condition. However, it is recognised that more effective communicative approaches could help address that behaviour (NICE, 2009). Therefore, this chapter examines how the nurse or midwife can implement communication skills to provide health education and enable positive behavioural change.

The importance of psychosocial care

In healthcare settings, nurses and midwives are the professions that spend the majority of time with patients and service users. They therefore regularly encounter people who may be acutely distressed at both the symptoms and implications of their illness. Psychosocial support is recognised as necessary in situations where people have experience of shock and/or trauma. Psychosocial support involves taking account of the psychological and social factors that are likely to be affected by a traumatic diagnosis and health experience.

The United Nations Commission on Human Rights (United Nations High Commission for Refugees, 2009, p. 10) defines the components of a psychosocial approach as follows: psychological components consist of 'mind, thoughts, feelings and behaviour'. These interact with the social components, namely 'interactions and relationships with others, environments, cultures and roles'.

Work with traumatised groups indicates that in order to build resilience and coping mechanisms, there is a need to take account of psychosocial factors. Agencies such as the United Nations point out that the issues outlined in the boxes above must also be addressed in addition to physical need. Psychological and social factors already existing in people's lives do not disappear with illness or trauma but will instead be affected by that illness/trauma. Therefore, all of these issues must be considered when delivering holistic care.

There are many examples of illness that can be both psychologically and physically challenging. Cancer care provides useful literature about the necessity of paying attention to the psychosocial needs of patients (Legg, 2011). In this section, cancer care is used as an example of the need to provide psychosocial care and demonstrates useful models for effective communication skills. Cancer is a potentially life-threatening condition, but it can be argued that the experiences of patients within this setting can shed light on the psychosocial needs of all patients facing challenging illness. Therefore, we propose that the examples cited here can be transferred to any acute or secondary care setting where patients are likely to be anxious and distressed.

Communicating with anxious or distressed patients

There is now recognition that a cancer diagnosis requires substantial psychological support, yet Sussman and Baldwin (2010) point out that lack of emotional care and adequate information is, all too often, the experience in the cancer patient's journey:

Evidence supports the effectiveness of services aimed at relieving the emotional distress that accompanies many chronic illnesses, including cancer, even in the case of debilitating depression and anxiety. Good evidence also underpins a number of interventions designed to help individuals adopt behaviours that can help them manage disease symptoms and improve their overall health. (Adler and Page, 2008, p. 7)

Many psychosocial issues can be addressed by simply being willing to ask the right questions and then referring to the appropriate support services. There are exemplars of good practice in psychosocial support in leading cancer centres (see e.g. www.royalmarsden. nhs.uk/your-care/support-services/psychological-care-and-counselling). Despite this, however, in some settings there is still a need for staff to develop their communication skills to effectively and supportively interact with patients.

Moore et al.'s (2013) systematic review of the impact of healthcare practitioners' communication on cancer patients highlighted the need for a high skill level in this area of care. The studies noted the psychological burden of a cancer diagnosis, necessitating practitioners to be able to simultaneously offer support and to provide clear and useful information. They pointed to the deleterious effects of ineffective communication where patients were left anxious and confused and were consequently less likely to adhere properly to prescribed treatment. In many cases, where patients felt dissatisfied and even resorted to litigation, it was professional communication rather than treatment options that was found to be lacking. The review also noted that experience and time are insufficient on their own, to guarantee that professionals are effective communicators, and concluded that communication training is essential.

One of the most worrying scenarios for many student nurses (as outlined by student nurses in the focus group advising content for this book) and also for some qualified nurses is the situation of the patient who has had the news of a worrying prognosis delivered and/or is clearly anxious about what is to happen. Offering the reassurance 'oh, everything will be OK' is unlikely to be helpful. The following extracts from Patient Opinion (www.patientopinion. org.uk/, 2015) (Patient stories 5.1 and 5.2) highlight the emotional impact for patients.

Patient story 5.1: Being empathic

The nurse, whose name I did not get sadly, was really lovely and accommodating. She gave me enough time to settle down and relax, which I really needed as I was so nervous I was in tears. She let my friend who came with me stay in the consulting room during the test. She really made it as easy an experience as possible for me.

If you ask me what experience any trainee doctor or nurse needs, it would be to shadow this nurse and see how she engaged with the patient and made things as easy as possible, and of course bantered with us all the while.

The demonstration of kindness and compassion, combined with effective and empathic communication skills, transformed a potentially frightening experience into a helpful clinical encounter. Compare this with Patient story 5.2.

Patient story 5.2: Lack of empathy

I am still devastated by my treatment at ******. When I talk about my time there I cry. It was one week ago that I was discharged. I arrived on the Saturday referred from ***** where I had been treated with care and compassion and left on the following Tuesday. I had two slipped discs and suspected CES and was in so much pain I couldn't walk at all. I was left in a nappy one time, I was helped to a commode during visiting time and had to use it behind the curtain whilst visitors could hear me. Patient dignity is last on the agenda. I was in pain and I was told that it was not protocol to use the pain meds that I had been given at *******, so I spent the first two days literally sobbing in pain and no one offered me anymore. Staff were curt, brief, often rude.

(www.patientopinion.org.uk/)

 Visit the Values Exchange website at http://sagecomms.vxcommunity.com for a broader discussion on this Patient story.

CRITICAL THINKING EXERCISE 5.1
EXPLAINING STAFF BEHAVIOUR

Could these experiences be any more contrasting? Take five minutes to consider what is going on. What explanations might be given as to why some staff can be kind and communicate well, whilst others reduce patients to tears?

Part 1 of this book explored listening, questioning and the development of an empathetic approach. It examined questions as to why nurses and other health professionals might be unable to respond helpfully to distressed patients. It is rarely the case that people enter these professions with the intention of being unkind to the people for whom they are supposed to care. However, a range of problems such as burnout, fear of saying the wrong thing and lacking the confidence to deal with emotion can result in behaviour that feels unkind to the patient.

Student story 5.1: Back to 'your worst fear'

In Chapter 1, we described how third-year students talked about doubting their abilities to talk with patients with terminal diagnoses. We discussed patient 'Ruth':

You arrive for your shift today, and your mentor says that Ruth has asked to see you specifically, although she doesn't know why. Approaching Ruth, she asks you for a "very large favour" and then bursts into tears. She explains that her results have revealed that she has a very rare form of an especially aggressive cancer, and it is now developed to such a stage that there is nothing that can be done except palliative care; the consultant has told her that she has about 10–20 days left. (extract from Chapter 1)

Ruth wants you, the student, to help her tell her family about her diagnosis. You want to help but you are still a student and need to remember your boundaries.

We suggest techniques that can help you communicate with patients such as 'Ruth'. It is more often feelings of incompetence and lack of confidence that prevent the nurse from demonstrating effective communication skills. Here, we take this further to examine useful techniques to enable nurses to respond in a helpful manner when faced with a difficult scenario. Jack et al. (2013) offer Simple Skills Secrets: this is a simple, yet effective model for any staff member, in any setting, when faced with unanswerable questions or being lost for words.

This model has been developed by those working within cancer care to enable the professional to respond and communicate helpfully in difficult circumstances. It was observed that some nurses were alarmed and unable to respond to patients who were clearly anxious and/or distressed. The model enables the nurse or midwife to acknowledge that whilst some situations cannot be easily resolved, patients should be able to voice concerns. It is not necessary for the healthcare practitioner to fix all situations but following a series of seven simple steps will enable the patient to express anxiety and plan their next move.

Simple Skills Secret

1. Patient gives cue
2. Healthcare professional asks open question
3. Listening and using silence
4. Encouraging
5. Summarising
6. Assisting the formation of the patient's own plan
7. Whilst resisting the urge to rush in with a solution

The Simple Skills Secret format invites the healthcare professional to respond to the patient's cue with an open question (remember open questions from Part 1?) – for example, 'What is concerning you?' in response to a verbal cue such as 'I'm concerned' or 'I'm a bit worried about…', or simply observing that the patient looks distressed or worried. There may well be silence at this point. The model stresses that allowing some time for silence is appropriate. Expect silence and do not be frightened of it. The ability to tolerate silence is a very effective attribute. Many rush to fill the void, whereas the void is an important aspect of communication in this situation. The use of silence gives the patient time to think about what they wish to say and it also shows that you have time to listen. It can encourage a patient to say more about their concerns.

It is then helpful to summarise and reflect back to the patient. Summarising helps the professional communicate and check for understanding:

'So what you are saying is that you are worried about...?'

Then, screening questions such as:

'Is there anything else that worries you?'

enables any additional and necessary information to be disclosed and allows for an 'unpeeling of the onion' (Jack et al., 2013, p. 1551).

The professional does not attempt to take over but then works collaboratively with the patient to make a plan (remember collaborative working from Part 1?):

'How would you like to take this forward?'

Collaborative decision making means that each person has an equal say. The model stresses that there is no need (in fact, it is discouraged) for the professional to rush in and rescue the situation. This simple, staged process enables the patient's voice to be heard but also stresses that the professional listens and takes their lead from the patient. As Jack et al. (2013) and Groves et al. (2014) note, health professionals are largely trained to 'do' and to feel that they must take the lead when these actions are not always the most appropriate response. There are situations that cannot be easily fixed but where it is imperative that the patient has the opportunity to express their feelings. The Simple Skills Secret stresses to the professional that it is acceptable and helpful to listen without feeling they must immediately resolve a problem.

_____ **CRITICAL THINKING EXERCISE 5.2** _____
A MINDFUL APPROACH

Using your thoughts, reflections and observations, now spend five minutes writing down your account of dealing with a patient with a distressing condition. What were your feelings about talking with the patient? How did the nurses respond to the patient? Try to identify where you observed a helpful or an unhelpful response. Describe the behaviours that made the response either helpful or unhelpful.

It is important to note that Simple Skills Secret is but one of a number of available models (see www.sageandthymetraining.org.uk for more resources). However, we highlight Simple Skills Secret as it is one that is being researched and evaluated with evidence emerging for its efficacy (Groves et al., 2014).

Communicating with those with long-term conditions to help change behaviour

Moving away from acute and secondary care, often to community and maternity care, it is recognised that health services need to improve communication and collaboration with patients and service users if the outcomes of living with long-term conditions are to be improved. Long-term conditions caused or exacerbated by unhealthy behaviour represent a major challenge for health services. These conditions can increase with age and, as is the case with other developed countries, the UK has an ageing population. However, Appleby (2013) points out a common misconception: the assumption that these older people will spend most of their older age in poor health and take up health resources. In fact, in developed countries the trend is for older people to spend their later years in better health and only use health resources in the period before death. It is not age that is the major issue for healthcare but the fact that more people are living with long-term conditions. Although the prevalence of long-term conditions rises with age, 'in absolute terms, there are more people with long-term conditions under the age of 65 than in older age groups' (Coulter et al., 2013, p. 3). As noted in Chapter 4, there is increasing concern at the effects of obesity in both parents and young children.

Barnett et al. (2012) found that 42% of the Scottish population had at least one long-term condition. Whereas those over 65 had multiple co-morbidities, these had developed 10–15 years earlier. Those most likely to be affected were also most likely to live in deprived circumstances. In England, it is estimated that the numbers of those with multiple conditions will increase from 1.9 million in 2008 to 2.9 million in 2018. Currently, it is the case that people with long-term conditions account for 70% of health and social care expenditure in England (House of Commons Health Committee, 2014). Therefore, conditions such as arthritis, diabetes, coronary heart disease, chronic kidney disease, mental health conditions, asthma, stroke, dementia, chronic obstructive pulmonary disease, hypertension and cancer make up the greatest challenge for health services. In addition, many of these people will have co-morbidities with combinations of these conditions.

This is a growing and possibly neglected issue in healthcare in developed countries. Although health behaviour is not causal in all conditions, it is the case in many and it certainly is a major factor in the management of long-term conditions. There is huge concern about the epidemic of diabetes and its associated complications, not least the fact that type 2 diabetes is becoming such a problem in relatively young people and children (Davies, 2014). Understanding of the health condition and the behaviour necessary to manage the condition is at least as important, if not more so, than medication (NICE, 2009). Although there is some early evidence that public health approaches influencing health behaviour are demonstrating improved outcomes in London, the results from much of the rest of England show the situation worsening (Public Health England, 2015).

A range of relatively simple tools has been in existence for some time to help individuals manage and change their health behaviour. Yet there seems to have been a reluctance by health services and health professionals to implement these. There may be a number of reasons for this: the development of a health service and professionals trained to 'do' not prevent; a human tendency to judge, 'nag' and 'victim blame' (Mason, 2005, p. 261). Mason notes: 'a common frustration expressed by health professionals is that their patients do not make the behaviour changes expected of them' (2005, p. 261). Possibly, this sounds familiar?

Rowan (2008, p. 402) provides an example: 'The 20-year-old female patient is eating potato crisps. She is visiting a medical centre for her cholesterol screening but it requires a 12 hour fast and she has been eating ... Is telling her off appropriate or useful? Should the situation be referred to senior staff?'

Mulherin et al. (2013) examined perceptions of care by obese, pregnant women and care providers' attitudes (including final-year midwifery students and medical students) towards obese pregnant women. They found that the women felt they had less positive care experiences and that significant numbers of care providers held stigmatising attitudes towards such service users.

Patient story 5.3: Pregnant and overweight

Then my family had brought me flowers and chocolate when they visited to which I was eating when the member of staff asked how much I weighed and could see I was overweight, to which I said it was nothing to do with them. The member of staff then said I shouldn't eat the chocolate, I was already big and hopefully my child wouldn't turn out big like me and walked away laughing saying poor baby a few times. (www.patientopinion.org.uk/)

Mold and Forbes (2011) also found evidence of stigma directed at overweight and pregnant women. This reflects societal views but, often, where professionals held these views, it was linked to concerns about risk management and feelings of a lack of competency in addressing weight management with service users.

CRITICAL THINKING EXERCISE 5.3
DO YOU JUDGE?

Using your thoughts, reflections and observations on your practice placement, now spend five minutes writing down your understanding of a person with a long-term condition such as diabetes and obesity. What were your feelings about the patient? What did you think should/could be done? Be honest.

Victim blaming and judging are unhelpful (if understandable) responses. Mason and Butler (2010) point out that although it is the patient who needs to change behaviour, poor communication with health professionals can make the situation worse. It is recognised that health services need to improve communication and collaboration with patients and service users if the experience of living with long-term conditions is to be tackled: 'Providing patients with long-term conditions with better information about their disease, choices for treatment and care pathways, and promoting self-care are hallmarks of high-quality care' (Department of Health, 2009, p. 2).

Public health approaches have long acknowledged the need to more effectively enable positive health behaviour. Policy makers and analysts now recognise this approach as becoming a necessity with general health services. NICE has current guidelines for services and practitioners working with those who would benefit from changing health behaviour (www.nice.org.uk/guidance/ph49) and is developing detailed guidance on long-term conditions. Diabetes and weight management is an issue of huge concern for health services at the moment.

Again, Patient Opinion (2015) provides an example in Patient story 5.4.

Patient story 5.4: Lack of help for weight loss

Visited the medical weight management department this morning as a new patient, as needed help with weight loss due to weight gain and having diabetes. Was extremely disappointed with the lack of empathy, concentration and questions asked by the doctor I saw. Felt like they were not really interested. I was not really asked about my medical conditions or what medication I am taking. I was just told they can't help me and they will discharge me from the department. It was a complete waste of my time despite having a referral from my GP and also the diabetic consultant at the hospital. Really disappointed with the level of service today, will be requesting not to be sent to this hospital in the future and will be advising others to do the same. Never been to a hospital that does not like to help people! (www.patientopinion.org.uk/, 2016)

Contrast that experience with the one in Patient story 5.5.

Patient story 5.5: help in weight management

I always find the diabetic day unit very encouraging and supportive as I cope with the unpleasant condition, even though my failure to control my weight over the years has contributed to me having this. It is also very helpful to see the same person **** each time I have an appointment. She can monitor the ups and down by seeing me over a period of time. It also means that I don't have to go through the saga of answering the same questions during each visit because yet another person has taken over my care. I am now losing weight which is very positive. (www.patientopinion.org.uk/, 2016)

And with the one in Patient story 5.6.

Patient story 5.6: encouragement to change behaviour

Attending my first appointment with healthy routes was not as bad as I imagined it would be. **** at the ***** Health Centre on ****** Road really put me at ease. I have Rheumatology arthritis and also osteoarthritis, so found myself gaining the pounds at a great rate due to medication and limited activity. I began to feel pretty down with myself, in fact totally losing self esteem. But I feel all that has changed, through giving that listening ear and all the positive encouragement and feedback from *** (So well done ***).

I have not lost a great deal of weight but what I have lost I have managed to keep off, again with encouragement. I have also started going swimming (only once a week) but I hope to increase this. I have always valued the time given to me at each appointment and never felt I was racing against the clock. But most importantly I was always being listened to. (www.patientopinion.org.uk/, 2016)

The type of communicative response encountered by patients makes a huge difference, not only to the patient's emotional state but also to their clinical outcomes.

There are many theoretical models and potential interventions associated with health behaviour change, however, as discussed in Part 1, motivational interviewing is an intervention that has been well researched and evaluated and demonstrates evidence of improved outcomes (Mason and Butler, 2010). In addition, it has been shown to be relatively simple to equip health professionals with these skills and they can be integrated into everyday practice. Therefore, this approach is selected for inclusion in this chapter.

Motivational interviewing is influenced by the trans-theoretical model of change proposed by Prochaska and DiClemente (1983, cited in Mason, 2005). This model (see Table 5.1) acknowledges that people will be naturally ambivalent about or resistant to change, despite knowing that their current behaviour harms their health. It also assumes that they are likely to relapse. This understanding that change has a natural process and that relapse is part of the process helps professionals work with, not against, patients.

Prochaska and DiClemente's stages of change

1. Pre-contemplation
2. Contemplation
3. Preparation
4. Action
5. Maintenance
6. Relapse

Recognition of the stage at which the patient is at enables the nurse or midwife to communicate most effectively. For example, very assertively discussing change, whilst the

Table 5.1   The transtheoretical model

Patient stage	Practitioner task
Precontemplation	Raise doubt and increase the patient's perception of the risks and problems with their current behaviour. Provide harm reduction strategies
Contemplation	Weigh up the pros and cons of change with the patient and work on helping them tip the balance by: • exploring ambivalence and alternatives • identifying reasons for change/risks of not changing • increasing the patient's confidence in their ability to change
Preparation and action	Clear goal setting – help the patient develop a realistic plan for making a change and to take steps toward change
Maintenance	Help the patient identify and use strategies to prevent relapse
Relapse	Help the patient renew the processes of contemplation and action without becoming stuck or demoralised

Source: Hall et al. (2012, p. 661)

Critical debate 5.1

Long-term conditions and a failure to address unhealthy behaviour are seen as one of the greatest threats to health in developed countries. Why is this the case? Do health professionals have a responsibility to do something about the situation?

Conclusion

Student nurses and midwives (and some qualified staff) are often concerned at the thought of being asked to provide psychological care for which they feel unprepared. They may avoid the patient rather than expose themselves to the risk of being in a situation where they feel out of control, especially when the prospect of a 'cure' is unlikely. In less acute settings, there is often frustration at the patient who will not alter their behaviour despite the fact that it is harming them. Both areas require addressing as the literature shows that patients want more psychological support and that clinical outcomes are improved when they receive this support. In many cases, nurses and midwives feel that unless they have considerable training in psychiatric techniques, they do not have the skills to support people. Although more training is always helpful, we argue that psychological support can be provided in relatively simple ways. As nurses and healthcare professionals, we can respond appropriately and supportively by listening, understanding a patient's perspective, and using simple yet effective techniques such as aspects of Simple Skills Secret and motivational interviewing. Ongoing training and research in parts of general healthcare demonstrate that systematic communicative techniques can be helpful to both the patient and the nurse in equipping both with effective coping mechanisms.

References

Adler, N. and Page, A. (2008) *Cancer Care for the Whole Patient: Meeting Psychosocial Health Needs*. Washington, DC: National Academies Press.

Appleby, J. (2013) *Spending on Health and Social Care over the Next 50 Years: Why Think Long Term?* London: Kings Fund.

Barnett, K., Mercer, S.W., Norbury, M., Watt, G., Wyke, S. and Guthrie, B. (2012) 'Epidemiology of multimorbidity and implications for health care, research, and medical education: a cross-sectional study', *The Lancet*, 380(9836): 37–43.

Coulter, A., Roberts, S. and Dixon, A. (2013) *Delivering Better Services to People with Long-term Conditions*. London: Kings Fund.

Davies, S. (2014) *Annual Report of the Chief Medical Officer, 2014 – The Health of the 51%: Women*. Available at: www.gov.uk/government/uploads/system/uploads/attachment_data/file/484383/cmo-report-2014.pdf

Department of Health (DoH) (2009) *Supporting People with Long-term Conditions*. London: The Stationery Office.

Groves, K., Jack, B., Baldry, C., O'Brien, M., Marley, K., Whelen, A. and Kirton, J. (2014) 'Simple skills secrets: a visual model of core communication skills for generic staff'. Paper presented at the 10th Palliative Care Congress, Harrogate International Centre, Harrogate, 12–14 March. Also in *British Medical Journal Supportive and Palliative Care*, 4.

Hall, K., Gibbe, T. and Lubman, D. (2012) 'Techniques for motivational interviewing', *Australian Family Physician*, 41(90): 660–7.

House of Commons Health Committee (2014) *Managing the Care of People with Long-term Conditions*. London: The Stationery Office.

Jack, B., Groves, K., Baldry, C., O'Brien, M., Marley, K., Whelan, A., et al. (2013) 'Communication for the nursing and healthcare workforce', *Nurse Education Today*, 33(12): 1550–6.

Legg, M. (2011) 'What is psychosocial care and how can nurses better provide it to adult oncology patients?', *Australian Journal of Advanced Nursing*, 28(3): 61–6.

Mason, P. (2005) 'Helping individuals change behaviour', in L. Ewles (ed.), *Key Topics in Public Health*. London: Churchill Livingstone. pp. 261–76.

Mason, P. and Butler, C. (2010) *Health Behavior Change: A Guide for Practitioners*. London: Elsevier.

Mold, F. and Forbes, A. (2011) 'Patients and professionals experiences and perspectives of obesity in health-care settings: a synthesis of current research', *Health Expectations*, 16: 119–142.

Moore, P., Mercado, R., Grez, M. and Lawrie, T. (2013) 'Communication skills training for professionals working with people who have cancer', *Cochrane Database Systematic Review*, 3: CD003751.

Mulherin, K., Miller, Y., Barlow, Diedrichs, F. and Thompson, R. (2013) 'Weight stigma in maternity care: women's experiences and care providers' attitudes', *BMC Pregnancy and Childbirth*, 13: 19.

National Institute for Health and Care Excellence (NICE) (2009) 'Self-care support for long-term conditions', Quality and Productivity case study, 27 November. Available at: www.nice.org.uk/savingsandproductivityandlocalpracticeresource?ci=http%3a%2f%2farms.evidence.nhs.uk%2fresources%2fQIPP%2f29520%3fniceorg%3dtrue (accessed 14 April 2016).

National Institute for Health and Care Excellence (NICE) (2015) 'Older people with social care needs and multiple long-term conditions'. NICE guidance NG22. Available at: www.nice.org.uk/Guidance/NG22 (accessed 14 April 2016).

Public Health England (2015) *Health Inequalities in London*. London: Public Health England. Available at: www.gov.uk/government/uploads/system/uploads/attachment_data/file/467805/Health_inequalities_in_London_Oct_15.pdf (accessed 12 March 2016).

Rowan, K. (2008) 'Monthly communication skill coaching for healthcare staff', *Patient Education and Counselling*, 71: 402–4.

Sussman, J. and Baldwin, L.M. (2010) 'The interface of primary and specialty care: from diagnosis through treatment', *Journal of the National Cancer Institute Monographs*, 40.

United Nations High Commission for Refugees (2009) 'Psychosocial intervention in complex emergencies: a framework for practice'. Working Paper, October. Available at: www.eldis.org/vfile/upload/1/document/1310/PWG_Framework_for_Practice.pdf

Useful websites

Patient Opinion home page – www.patientopinion.org.uk/

Public Health England home page – www.gov.uk/government/organisations/public-health-england

Stephen Rollnick et al.'s 'Motivational interviewing in health care' – http://web.vu.lt/mf/r.viliuniene/files/2014/10/Motivational-Interviewing-in-Health-Care.-Helping-Patients-Change-Behavior.pdf

Stephen Rollnick's consultancy and training site – www.stephenrollnick.com/

The King's Fund on managing long-term conditions – www.kingsfund.org.uk/projects/gp-inquiry/management-long-term-conditions

The Royal Marsden NHS Foundation Trust on psychological care and counselling – www.royalmarsden.nhs.uk/your-care/support-services/psychological-care-and-counselling

UCL's Health Behaviour Research Centre home page – www.ucl.ac.uk/hbrc

To access further resources related to this chapter, visit the Values Exchange website at http://sagecomms.vxcommunity.com

6

Communication for Mental Health: Understanding the Effects of Stigma

Graeme Reid

• • • • • • • • • • • • Learning Objectives • • • • • • • • • • •

By the end of this chapter, you will have developed an understanding of:

- the prevalence and persistence of stigma attached to mental health conditions
- avoiding stigmatising communication and behaviours within general settings
- looking past diagnoses to achieve person-centred care within mental health services.

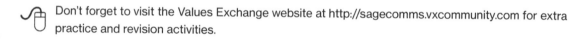 Don't forget to visit the Values Exchange website at http://sagecomms.vxcommunity.com for extra practice and revision activities.

• •

Introduction

There are no special tips or techniques to communicating with service users with mental health problems with which this chapter could aim to equip the reader beyond those already covered in the book. This is because, on a skills level, effective communication with a service user with mental health problems bears little difference to communicating with any other service user. The same Simple Skills Secrets highlighted in the previous chapter – recognising cues, open questioning, use of silence, etc. – continue to apply. As discussed throughout this book, the capacity to empathise is a cornerstone to therapeutic engagement with service users, yet when it comes to the concept of mental health conditions, misconceptions, ignorance and negative beliefs continue to endure, even (and in some cases, especially) amongst mental health professionals. Instead, this chapter aims to explore how stigma – the antithesis of empathy – impacts on the delivery of care to service users with mental health conditions, within both general and psychiatric settings.

Student contributors to this book from the general, child and learning disability field reflected on how – when they discovered that as part of their education they were to under-take a brief 'insight' placement within a mental health setting – they felt 'afraid' of what was to come. Studies have shown that universities in several countries have struggled to attract applicants to mental health nursing for similar reasons (Thongpriwan et al., 2015). This fear of the 'mentally ill' has run deep within society for centuries and has clearly left its mark. Through discussion of how stigma is experienced by service users and at times perpetuated within healthcare environments, it is hoped that the reader will develop an awareness of how to safeguard against and tackle stigma within the working environment, and develop and maintain positive therapeutic relationships with service users.

CRITICAL THINKING EXERCISE 6.1
MINDFULNESS

Using your thoughts, reflections and observations on your practice placement, now spend five minutes writing down your understanding of a person with a mental health condition. How did you feel? What were your concerns about interacting with people with mental health issues? Did meeting people with mental illness change your perceptions? If so, how? Be honest.

What is stigma?

Before discussing the far-reaching ramifications of stigma in how nurses communicate with service users, it is important first to clarify the concept. The word itself derives from Greek origin, referring to a mark or tattoo that was burnt onto the skin of crimi-nals in order to visibly identify them as such and shame them publically. Broadly speaking, 'stigma' in contemporary usage applies to the social phenomenon whereby a set of discriminatory beliefs about a group of people – be it based on ethnicity, sexuality, class, etc. – is ingrained and enacted within a given culture.

Sociological theory around stigma was pioneered by Erving Goffman in the 1960s. Goffman (1963: 3) formulated stigma as 'an attribute that is [seen to be] deeply dis-crediting' that functions to reduce the individual from 'a whole and usual person' to one who is 'tainted'. Much of the literature that followed Goffman's seminal text centred on the individual's experience of stigma, particularly how stigma was internalised to affect a person's emotions and shape their behaviours. This led to the concept of self-stigma, whereby individuals, as part of their development into adulthood, become aware of society's low opinion of them (for whatever given trait or behaviour they possess), leading to low self-esteem and a discouragement in pursuing life goals (Corrigan et al., 2009).

Student story 6.1: John (part 1)

I was shocked when on placement to meet a 25-year-old man, John, with a diagnosis of bipolar disorder who said he would 'rather stay in hospital' indefinitely than return home and receive input from the community team. Due to the onset of his illness, John had failed to complete

(Continued)

(Continued)

his third year at university. He blamed himself for this and regularly stated 'I've ruined my life'; despite still showing a passionate interest in American history, he dismissed suggestions that he could ever resume his studies. The reason why he did not want to return home was a fear that friends and neighbours would become aware that he was being visited by mental health professionals and that 'they would know I'm ****** in the head'.

 Visit the Values Exchange website at http://sagecomms.vxcommunity.com for a broader discussion on this Patient story.

Many theorists in the wake of Goffman felt that this line of thinking, whilst still relevant, implied a responsibility on the part of the individual being stigmatised. Once the domain of social psychologists, theory around stigma has evolved considerably with the input of anthropologists and other disciplines to broaden the emphasis outward and identify the mechanisms within society which give rise to stigma. As such, it is now widely accepted that stigma is comprised of a number of social processes interacting. This is exemplified by the model of stigma provided by Link and Phelan (2001).

Component model of stigma

Link and Phelan (2001) identify five components of stigma:

- labelling
- stereotyping
- separation
- status loss
- discrimination.

Labelling involves the identification of human differences, elevated to social significance within a given group or culture. As Link and Phelan note, there are myriad superficial ways in which individuals differ from one another – eye colour, height, shoe size, for example – but most of these are considered unimportant socially. Why is it then that other differences – skin colour, sexuality, body shape – seem to matter so much? It is noted that the labelling process involves an oversimplification of difference, commonly into a binary formulation. For example, 'black' or 'white' and 'straight' or 'gay' – we live in a society which will still frequently identify mixed-race people as 'black' and bisexual people as 'gay', despite protests for less rigid thinking.

Labelling is accompanied by **stereotyping**. Link and Phelan define stereotypes as 'a set of undesirable characteristics' applied, in most cases, automatically and pre-consciously in response to a given label. The application of labels and stereotypes involves a process of **separation**, or 'us' vs. 'them' thinking, whereby the identified undesirability of a group becomes the rationale for believing they are fundamentally different from those who escape the label. The separation process functions to devalue the person or group hierarchically, so that they experience a **loss of status** in the eyes of the stigmatiser. This process is exemplified at its worst throughout history in the enabling of slavery and genocide. In terms of historical approaches to mental illness, the process is demonstrable in the removal of the mentally unwell from 'decent' society, leading to routine incarceration in asylums where individuals did not receive treatment (Foerschner, 2010).

The act of **discrimination** against a stigmatised person or group is distinguished in two forms by Link and Phelan: **individual discrimination**, whereby one person discriminates against another in an overt way (and is the reason why details such as age, gender, ethnicity, sexual preference and religion are obscured in most job applications these days); and **structural discrimination**. This latter category refers to institutional practices that function to disadvantage an identified group on a broad level; for example, it continues to be argued that on both a national (Centre for Economic Performance, 2012) and an international level, structural discrimination results in significant disparity between funding for mental health services and that for physical conditions (Zimmerman and Gazarian, 2014).

How is mental health stigmatised within society?

Although stigma exists around some physical health conditions – such as obesity and sexually transmitted diseases – the stigmatisation of mental health is demonstrably more ingrained within our culture. Despite having come a long way from the Draconian, separationist approach to mental illness, the crude dichotomy between 'madness' and 'sanity' persists, and the pejorative language of 'lunatics' and 'maniacs' which derives from archaic psychiatry remains in common colloquial usage. The tabloid press can regularly be seen to propagate a language of fear and otherness in their depiction of mental illness. As recently as 2015, when it was discovered that the Germanwings co-pilot Andreas Lubitz – who intentionally crashed a plane into the French Alps – had a past history of depression (notably, not a diagnosis that is otherwise commonly portrayed as dangerous), the UK front pages were emblazoned with headlines such as 'MADMAN IN COCKPIT' (*Sun* newspaper, 27 March 2015). Other examples of this can be seen below:

- ARMED AND DANGEROUS: PUBLIC AT RISK AS MENTAL PATIENTS ESCAPE THE CARE NET (*Daily Express*, 1998) – grossly exaggerating research findings that 6 out of 23 patients with schizophrenia carried weapons during psychotic episodes (Ferriman, 2000)
- GET THE VIOLENT CRAZIES OFF OUR STREETS (*The Daily News*, 1999) – a New York paper warns of 'the violence of the mentally ill' after a woman is attacked by a man with no known history of mental illness (Kelley, 2000)
- BONKERS BRUNO LOCKED UP (*Sun*, 2003) – reporting on boxer Frank Bruno being sectioned under the Mental Health Act (Gibson, 2003)
- INSANE! INSIDE BRITNEY'S TRAGIC FREEFALL INTO MADNESS – Britney Spears' experience with bipolar disorder gets sensationalised by *Star* magazine, 2008
- 1,200 KILLED BY MENTAL PATIENTS (*Sun*, 2013) – irresponsibly skewing the data from an annual report by the University of Manchester, and overlooking the statistic that 95% of homicides in England and Wales were committed 'by individuals who had not been diagnosed with a mental health problem' (Chalabi, 2013).

The mental health diagnosis which has most often been linked by the press and within popular culture with notions of violence and unpredictability has been schizophrenia. It is a commonly held misconception that schizophrenia amounts to a 'Jekyll and Hyde' syndrome, characterised by a 'split personality' where a seemingly 'sane' person has a secret, dangerous side (McNally, 2007). Furthermore, as Stuart (2008) notes, 'the general public uses schizophrenia as a paradigm for mental illness', using the term (or its abridged 'schizo') to describe any unusual or disorganised behaviours. The difference between common perceptions and the lived experience of schizophrenia can be seen in the popular blog 'The Secret Schizophrenic'.

Patient story 6.1: The secret schizophrenic

Before I started to get ill, I most likely thought the same as the popular understanding of schizophrenia: that it is a multiple personality disorder with violent tendencies, something that you would see in the news about murderers. So, once you receive that diagnosis, you start to feel like the popular opinion is against you. (The Secret Schizophrenic blog at www.time-to-change.org.uk, 2012)

 Visit the Values Exchange website at http://sagecomms.vxcommunity.com for a broader discussion on this Patient story.

Fighting stigma

One of the most unfortunate effects of mental health stigma within society is that individuals who are experiencing or are at risk of developing mental health problems may refrain from accessing support due to the level of denial or shame felt. In 2015, in response to a dramatic spike in male suicide rates over the last decade, and bolstered by research evidence that men were reticent to speak about mental distress or low mood (Pedersen and Paves, 2014), the Campaign Against Living Miserably (CALM) was launched (Figure 6.1). In its promotional material, the campaign recognised the intersection between mental health stigma and gender stereotypes, portraying 'manly' clichés as potentially life-threatening in order to persuade men to access professional support.

Since 2009, the charities MIND and Rethink Mental Illness have been running their 'Time to Change' campaign which uses the slogan 'let's end mental health discrimination'. Amongst many achievements, the Time to Change campaign has worked alongside organisations from all sectors in order to improve policy and reduce discrimination in the workplace; involved schools to dispel misconceptions about mental health amongst children and young people; and provided funding grants to pilot a number of community projects nationwide designed and organised by people with mental health problems (www.time-to-change.org.uk).

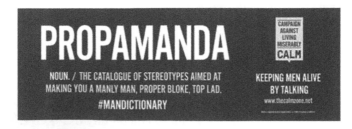

Figure 6.1   Propamanda

Reproduced with permission from CALM (thecalmzone.net)

The increase in anti-discrimination campaigns has occurred in parallel to the increased centrality of a *recovery-focused model of care* within mental health provision. The concept of 'recovery' as used in contemporary NHS policy has shifted away from the more traditional concept of eradicating symptoms and quieting distress to incorporate the psychosocial principles of holistic and collaborative care. The charity Rethink Mental Illness identifies recovery as 'the building of a meaningful and satisfying life, as defined by the person themselves, whether or not there are ongoing symptoms or problems' (Bora, 2012).

Avoiding stigmatising communication within general settings

How is mental health stigmatised within healthcare?

Despite the increased emphasis within healthcare services and nursing education on recovery and collaborative care, there remains a pronounced dichotomy between mental and physical health. Student contributors to this book who were undertaking studies in the general nursing field reported that they felt they were not receiving adequate training around mental health and even observed stigmatising attitudes espoused by their lecturers, both factors which they felt affected their confidence when encountering individuals with mental health needs in practice.

The need for more comprehensive training around mental health conditions is a common finding in studies of nursing communication within general settings. Given that Accident & Emergency departments are a frequent point of entry into the mental health system for many patients, a number of studies have been conducted within this setting, and many stigmatising behaviours from nursing staff have been recorded.

A common issue found was the risk of diagnostic overshadowing; i.e. assuming that the patient's pre-documented mental health problem is the true source of his or her distress and overlooking the physical problem. In one example, a man with a diagnosis of schizophrenia presented to A&E after a serious fall – the staff attributed his 'strange' behaviour to his schizophrenia and he was admitted to a mental health ward. The following day it was discovered that he had in fact suffered a brain injury and required urgent admission to neurosurgery in order to stop internal bleeding (Institute of Psychiatry, 2012).

Other studies have highlighted the dominant association of mental health with violence or aggression. Expectations of volatile and abusive behaviour in staff in an emergency department have led to outright avoidance of patients with mental health problems, resulting in longer waiting times for these patients (Broadbent et al., 2004). Furthermore, where aggression or frustration with the environment has been displayed by individuals, there have been examples found of staff deliberately engineering longer waiting times as a means of punishment for this behaviour (Kerrison and Chapman, 2007). Of course, by extending patients' time spent in the waiting room, aggressive behaviours have been exacerbated and increased the use of chemical interventions.

It is not just within accident and emergency departments that patients with mental health needs appear. There is a high statistical co-morbidity between mental health problems and long-term physical conditions, notably diabetes and schizophrenia for example, and it is important to remember that a patient with mental health problems can have just as much insight into their physical condition as any other patient. Stensrud et al. (2014) provide a set of six evidence-based skills to employ in interactions with patients with mental health issues in general settings and also provide examples of helpful and empowering responses (Table 6.1).

Table 6.1   Six evidence-based skills to employ in interactions with patients with mental health issues and examples of helpful responses

Skills	Examples
Explore emotions (be sensitive to and explore the patient's hints, concerns and emotions)	'You say it's been difficult for you lately...?' 'Can you tell me more about that?'
Respond empathically (be explicitly empathic to emotional content)	'I understand you worry about cancer' 'That must be hard for you'
Explore the patient's perspective and understanding	'What do you think might be the cause of your problem?'
Provide insight into possible cause–effect relations of the problem	'When you ruminate and have trouble sleeping, that could influence your headache too'
Explore resources (assess the patient's resources and strengths)	'You must be quite resilient to be able to deal with this for so long' 'Have you found any ways that alleviate the pain?'
Promote coping and empowerment	'Maybe it's possible to use that strategy in this situation as well'

Source: Stensrud et al. (2014)

It can be seen that the communicative strategies suggested by Stresnud et al. consist of simply responding to the patient with a co-existing mental health condition in the same caring and compassionate way a nurse would with any other patient. The only thing that prevents this occurring is the lingering assumption that the mentally unwell patient is fundamentally different.

Looking past diagnoses to achieve person-centred care within mental health services

Stigma within mental health services: borderline personality disorder

Paradoxically, mental health professionals can be as guilty as perpetuating stigma as any other healthcare professional. One of the most stigmatised groups within mental health services is those with personality disorder – particularly borderline personality disorder (BPD). Although public misconceptions and discrimination against schizophrenia and depression have been the focus of pushback from mental health charities in recent years, 'personality disorder' remains a rather under-discussed condition in the media, so much so that the layman may not be as familiar with the term as with other conditions. Within the terrain of mental health services, however, it is perhaps the most stigmatised. The following section will outline why this is the case, identify specific stereotyping of the disorder that occurs within services, and suggest ways in which practitioners can be mindful of this in order to enhance their relationships with patients.

The *Diagnostic and Statistical Manual of Mental Disorder* (DSM) IV lists the following criteria for borderline personality disorder:

- Uses extreme measures to avoid real or imagined abandonment
- Volatile relationships with others that can alternate between admiration and depreciation
- Identify issues with an unstable self-esteem
- Irresponsibility in at least two potentially harmful areas
- Suicidal behaviours; gestures or threats
- Self-mutilating behaviour
- Mood fluctuation with noticeable, rapid changes
- Persistent feelings of emptiness
- Inappropriate, extreme or hard to control anger
- Short lasting stress-related paranoia or dissociation. (DSM-IV)

Borderline personality disorder as a concept has remained quite difficult to pin down. The term 'borderline' was coined by Adolph Stern in 1938 (Bateman and Norcross, 2011) to describe presentation that was neither 'psychotic' nor 'neurotic' but somewhere in between. This ambiguity can be seen to have persisted over time as 'borderline personality disorder' has proven difficult to define. As recently as 2013, in the advent of the publication of the *Diagnostic and Statistical Manual of Mental Disorders*, 5th edition (DSM-5), there was controversy over the diagnostic criteria for borderline personality disorder, with many critics calling for radical changes to be made, in large part on the grounds that the established diagnosis reinforced stigma. Ultimately, the update made only minor amendments to the diagnostic criteria but significantly it recognised – for the first time – personality disorder as a serious mental illness under the same category as schizophrenia and bipolar disorder. Above is shown the DSM-IV criteria which has been used since 2000. This elusiveness in terms of diagnosis has run parallel to the misconception that BPD is an 'untreatable' condition, effectively making the diagnosis a life-sentence. Recent studies have shown that patients with BPD are 'as treatable' as patients with depressive disorders (Gunderson et al., 2009). Despite such recent findings however, BPD continues to be widely regarded as a 'dustbin diagnosis', and harmful stereotypes about those diagnosed with BPD continue to abound.

'Difficult patients'

As identified earlier in the chapter, labelling and separation are major components of the stigma process. Within mental health services, language used commonly amongst professionals has been observed that demonstrates these components in action. Sulzer (2015) describes how the concept of 'the difficult patient' has been prevalent within psychiatry since at least the 1970s, most frequently being applied to patients who were 'hard to work with' or did not appear to respond to treatment. Sulzer argues that the complex history of defining and treating borderline personality disorder has contributed to ingrained expectations that a patient bearing the diagnosis (or 'label') will be inherently 'difficult'.

Patients with borderline personality disorder are also commonly dismissed by nursing staff as 'manipulative', 'demanding' and 'time-wasters' (Bonnington and Rose, 2014). These stereotypes appear to have risen primarily in response to the propensity of BPD patients towards self-harming or 'destructive' behaviours which are not perceived to be 'genuine' in intent but merely a gambit to secure nurses' attention or achieve a desired effect. However, when patients bearing a different diagnosis (schizophrenia or bipolar disorder, for example) exhibit similar behaviours it has been found that nurses respond more empathetically. Woollaston and Hixenbaugh (2008) argue that this occurs due to BPD lacking clearly demarcated signs and symptoms of distress (such as auditory and visual hallucinations, paranoid beliefs) and, as a result, nurses believing that the person with BPD is more 'in control' of their behaviour. Although 'uses extreme measures to avoid real or imagined abandonment' is a recognised criterion in diagnosing BPD, it is not generally considered a 'symptom' of an illness in the same way that hallucinations or low mood are.

The instability in interpersonal relationships characteristic of BPD – the alternation between 'admiration and depreciation' – often manifests itself in the patient rejecting care from staff. This is said to confound the caregiver role, stirring up complex emotional responses within the nurse including a sense of hopelessness. Particularly in the case of working with patients with personality disorder, reflective practice and clinical supervision are advised; it is the responsibility of the nurse to monitor their own behaviour, especially if they are going to criticise that of their patients (Houghton and Ousley, 2004).

Student story 6.2: John (part 2)

Although John had been officially diagnosed with bipolar disorder, over the course of his admission this was questioned by nursing staff, one of whom stated that 'he's not unwell, it's all personality related'. In the days approaching his discharge from hospital, his anxiety levels were observed to be escalating, he was utilising his unescorted leave less frequently, and his demeanour was increasingly described as 'hostile'. Towards the end of a shift one evening, John appeared at the nursing office and banged on the window; his face was bloody with a split lip and he shouted 'I've beat myself up, send me back to PICU'. He walked away from the staff who approached him. One of the nurses dismissed this as 'behavioural' and said 'he'll be out of here soon anyway'. Other staff members approached him shortly afterwards and offered to listen to what he was going through. It transpired that, underlying his anger and distress, were his concerns about care in the community; the staff were able to allay these fears by discussing with him alternative options for follow-up care, so that he did not have to receive visits at home. It occurred to me that, had these staff members not intervened in this way, John's recovery may have encountered a set-back. It also occurred to me that, had someone discussed John's wishes with him days earlier, when his increased anxiety and hostility were first reported, this 'behaviour' may have been avoided.

CRITICAL THINKING EXERCISE 6.2
MINDFULNESS

Using your thoughts, reflections and observations on your practice placement, now spend five minutes writing down your experience with a 'difficult patient'. How did you feel? How did you respond? Be honest.

How can you communicate in non-stigmatising ways?

It is worthwhile when working with 'difficult patients' – whether they have a BPD diagnosis or not – to bear in mind the long-standing concept of **unconditional positive regard,** introduced by psychotherapist Carl Rogers. Unconditional positive regard is said to be 'achieved by accepting others as individuals who are entitled to respect and care' (Gamble and Curthoys, 2004). The psychotherapeutic and patient-centred principles of Rogers' approach both complement the recovery model of care and counteract the prevalence of stigma by acknowledging the individuality and personhood of the patient beyond the labels and stereotypes.

Swift (2009) identified the need for nurses to focus on 'questioning and understanding rather than on blaming and punishing'. In addition to the components of stigma addressed earlier, Link and Phelan also emphasised that discriminatory actions always require a context of power in which to be enacted (Link and Phelan, 2001). John Heron's Six Category Intervention Analysis provides a useful framework which can help nurses monitor how their communication with patients may be reinforcing or relying on this power dynamic. Heron defines an intervention as 'an identifiable piece of verbal and/or non-verbal behaviour that is part of the practitioner's service to the client' (2001: 3), thus demonstrating how every interaction that occurs – no matter how seemingly minor – between staff and service user contributes to the therapeutic relationship. Heron divided the six communication styles identified under two categories – authoritative interventions (whereby the nurse takes a more directive role in the relationship) and facilitative interventions (which aim to minimise the power dynamic in the staff-patient relationship and encourage autonomy) (see Table 6.2).

Although not all authoritative interventions are stigmatising, stigmatising behaviours from nurses often invoke authority. Collaborative communication cannot be achieved by reliance on purely authoritative interventions; the accomplished, non-stigmatising nurse will achieve an adept balance of both styles of intervention, utilising the six sub-categories intuitively and effectively within interpersonal communication (Burnard and Morrison, 2005).

Table 6.2   Heron's six category intervention

Authoritative	
Prescriptive	Offer advice, make suggestions, give instruction
Informative	Give information, impart knowledge, provide psychoeducation
Confronting	Challenge the person's thoughts and behaviours, reflect back statements and actions
Facilitative	
Cathartic	Enable the expression of emotions and fears, empathise with person
Catalytic	Ask questions to encourage new ways of considering something, encourage person to generate new ideas or strategies
Supportive	Offer support, make person feel valued, praise achievements

Source: Heron (2001)

Student (and patient) story 6.3: 'Life-changing care'

I have suffered from low mood and crippling (social) anxiety since I was a child. Aside from a brief period talking to a mental health nurse as a teenager, my problems were always dismissed by my GP at home, with years of visits only ever getting me the same printed pages of self-help and eventually the lowest dose of propranolol (beta blocker) because I would be physically shaking with nerves every university seminar I attended. I would leave the surgery tearful, feeling like a stupid child; embarrassed to have wasted their time with such an apparently trivial problem. When I moved to ******to train as a nurse myself I signed up with the ***** Student Medical Practice. I can honestly say that for three years I received the best quality treatment and care I could have wished for.

Despite still training as a GP, I will never forget the registrar I spoke to and her kindness and professionalism; immediately assessing me for anxiety/depression (my anxiety score was in the 'severe' range), talking through all the medical and psychological options I had and then asking what I would like to do. Since being listened to, having my problem acknowledged and starting on an SSRI that day my life has honestly changed. (www.patientopinion.org.uk/, 2015)

 Visit the Values Exchange website at http://sagecomms.vxcommunity.com for a broader discussion on this Student (and patient) story.

Critical debate 6.1

What do you really think about mental health/illness? Should all nurses be able to communicate effectively with people with mental health problems? If not, why not? If so, what needs to change in nurse education?

Conclusion

This chapter has stressed that there are no special secrets to communicating with people with mental illness. The same techniques that apply to other groups of people, particularly when distressed by illness, apply to those with mental health problems. However, understanding of the context of communicating with people with mental health problems is essential to good communication within mental health. Therefore, this chapter concentrated on stigma as people with mental illness are possibly the most stigmatised (certainly amongst the most marginalised) group in society. The health professional is invited to look at the definition of stigma and consider how stigma affects the perception of the stigmatised person or group. Communication is improved by understanding the effects of stigma and taking action to combat and tackle stigmatising behaviour in ourselves. Self-awareness as to how we communicate, monitoring and identifying our communicative styles, helps the professional to develop non-discriminatory and collaborative interaction with mental health service users.

References

Bateman, A.W. and Norcross, J.C. (2011) *History of Psychotherapy: Continuity and Change* (2nd edn, edited by VandenBos, G.R. and Freedheim, D.K.), pp. 588–600. Washington, DC: American Psychological Association.

Bonnington, O. and Rose, D. (2014) 'Exploring stigmatisation among people diagnosed with either bipolar disorder or borderline personality disorder: a critical realist analysis', *Social Science and Medicine*, 123: 7–17.

Bora, R. (2012) *Empowering People: Coaching for Mental Health Recovery*. Rethink Mental Illness. Available at: www.rethink.org/resources/e/empowering-people-coaching-for-mental-health-reco very (accessed 3 March 2016).

Broadbent, M., Jarman, H. and Berk, M. (2004) 'Emergency department mental health triage scales improve outcomes', *Journal of Evaluation in Clinical Practice*,10 (1): 57–62.

Burnard, P. and Morrison, P. (2005) 'Nurses' perceptions of their interpersonal skills', *Nurse Education Today*, 25(8): 612–17.

Centre for Economic Performance (2012) *How Mental Illness Loses Out in the NHS*. Available at: http://cep.lse.ac.uk/pubs/download/special/cepsp26.pdf

Chalabi, M. (2013) 'The Sun says 1,200 people have been killed by "mental patients" – is it true?', *The Guardian*, 7 October. Available at: www.theguardian.com/society/reality-check/2013/oct/07/ sun-people-killed-mental-health-true (accessed 3 March 2016).

Corrigan, P., Larson, J. and Rusch, N. (2009) 'Self-stigma and the "why-try" effect: impact on life goals and evidence-based practices', *World Psychiatry*, 8: 75–81.

Ferriman, A. (2000) 'The stigma of schizophrenia', *BMJ: British Medical Journal*, 320(7233): 522.

Foerschne, A. (2010) *A History of Mental Illness: From Skull Drills to Happy Pills*, Vol. 2, No. 09: p.1.

Gamble, C. and Curthoys, J. (2004) 'Psychosocial interventions', in Norman, I. and Ryrie, I. (eds), *The Art and Science of Mental Health Nursing: A Textbook of Principles and Practice*. Maidenhead: Open University Press.

Gibson, O. (2003) 'Sun on the ropes over "Bonkers Bruno" story', *The Guardian*, 23 September. Available at: www.theguardian.com/media/2003/sep/23/pressandpublishing.mentalhealth

Goffman, E. (1963) *Stigma: Notes on the Management of Spoiled Identity*. New York: Prentice-Hall.

Gunderson, J. (2009) *Borderline Personality Disorder: A Clinical Guide*. Washington, DC: American Psychiatric Publishing, Inc.

Heron, J. (2001) *Helping the Client: A Practical, Creative Guide*. Thousand Oaks, CA: Sage.

Houghton, S. and Ousley, L. (2004) 'The person with a personality disorder', in Norman, I. and Ryrie, I. (eds), *The Art and Science of Mental Health Nursing: A Textbook of Principles and Practice* (Chapter 21). Maidenhead: Open University Press.

Institute of Psychiatry (2012) *Why People with Mental Health Problems might not Get the Treatment They Need in A&E*. Available at: mentalhealthcare.org.uk/media/downloads/accident_and_emer gency.pdf

Kelley, T. (2000) 'Suspect pleads not guilty in brick attack on woman', *New York Times*, 8 January. Available at: www.nytimes.com/2000/01/08/nyregion/suspect-pleads-not-guilty-in-brick-attack-on-woman.html

Kerrison, S. and Chapman, R. (2007) 'What general emergency nurses want to know about mental health patients presenting to their emergency department', *Accident and Emergency Nursing*, 15: 48–55.

Link, B. and Phelan, J. (2001) 'Conceptualizing stigma', *Annual Review of Sociology*, 27: 363–85.

McNally, K. (2007) 'Schizophrenia as split personality/Jekyll and Hyde: the origins of the informal usage in the English language', *Journal of the History of the Behavioural Sciences*, 43(1): 69–79.

Pedersen, E. and Paves, A. (2014) 'Comparing perceived public stigma and personal stigma of mental health treatment seeking in a young adult sample', *Psychiatry Research*, 219(1): 143–50.

Stensrud, T., Gulbrandson, P., Mjaaland, T., Skretting, S. and Finset, A. (2014) 'Improving communication in general practice when mental health issues appear: piloting a set of six evidence-based skills', *Patient Education and Counseling*, 95: 69–75.

Stuart, H. (2008) 'Fighting the stigma caused by mental disorders: past perspectives, present activities, and future directions', *World Psychiatry*, 7(3): 185–8.

Sulzer, S. (2015) 'Does "difficult patient" status contribute to de facto demedicalization? The case of borderline personality disorder', *Social Science & Medicine*, 142: 82–9.

Swift, E. (2009) 'The efficacy of treatments for borderline personality disorder', *Mental Health Practice*, 13(4): 30–3.

Thongpriwan, V., Leuck, S., Powell, R., Young, S., Schuler, S. and Hughes, R. (2015) 'Undergraduate nursing students' attitudes toward mental health nursing', *Nurse Education Today*, 35: 948–53.

Woollaston, K. and Hixenbaugh, P. (2008) 'Destructive whirlwind: nurses' perceptions of patients diagnosed with borderline personality disorder', *Journal of Psychiatric and Mental Health Nursing*, 15(9): 703–9.

Zimmerman, M. and Gazarian, D. (2014) 'Is research on borderline personality disorder underfunded by the National Institute of Health?', *Psychiatry Research*, 220: 941–4.

Useful websites

CALM: Campaign Against Living Miserably home page – thecalmzone.net

Mind home page – www.mind.org.uk/

Rethink Mental Illness home page – www.rethink.org/

Time to Change home page – www.time-to-change.org.uk

Young Minds: Stigma – A Review of the Evidence –www.youngminds.org.uk/assets/0000/1324/stigma-review.pdf

 To access further resources related to this chapter, visit the Values Exchange website at http://sagecomms.vxcommunity.com

7

Communicating with People with Cognitive Deficits

Jean Shapcott

• • • • • • • • • • • • Learning Objectives • • • • • • • • • • • •

By the end of this chapter, you will have developed an understanding of:

- communicating with people with reduced intellectual capacity such as learning disabilities and head injury
- communicating with people who have dementia.

Don't forget to visit the Values Exchange website at http://sagecomms.vxcommunity.com for extra practice and revision activities.

• •

Introduction

The complex dynamics of communication which are an integral part of the nurse–patient relationship is significantly influenced by the ability of each party to communicate (Morris and Morris, 2010). People communicate their needs, wishes and feelings as a means of maintaining their quality of life and preserving a sense of identity (Jootun and McGhee, 2011), and when this ability is compromised it is important that the nurse demonstrates sensitivity and encourages the person to communicate in whatever way suits them best.

For any individual, limited intellectual capacity can have a profound effect on their ability to communicate. Whether the problems were present from birth, acquired through a brain injury or the result of cognitive decline, a person's communicative style and effectiveness will inevitably be affected to some degree. It would be all too easy to list different communication strategies in some form of hierarchy in which spoken and written language is considered more important and significant than, for example, signs or symbols (Pardoe, 2011). Nurses are generally familiar with and use spoken language without a second thought, but this may not be of any value when communicating with individuals in this category.

This chapter will explore strategies that can be used by nurses to communicate with people who have diminished intellectual capacity. As well as considering the application of specific verbal and non-verbal strategies, the value of really getting to know individuals and their communicative styles and patterns will be considered within person-centred communication. The concept of Total Communication, a system which is concerned with exploring all aspects of communication in order to discover what works best for the individual, will be addressed alongside Augmentative and Alternative Communication strategies. When someone experiences a decline in their cognitive ability, maybe as a result of a neurological degenerative disease or dementia, it is equally important to practise person-centred techniques, some of which, such as the use of Talking Mats (www.talkingmats.com/), are the same as those used with people with intellectual disability, whilst others, for example empathic curiosity, reflect the individual's previous abilities and life experiences.

Communicating with people with intellectual disability

Intellectual (or learning) disability can be defined as an impairment which started before adulthood, has a lasting effect on development and is characterised by a significantly reduced ability to understand new or complex information or learn new skills and a reduced ability to cope independently (Pardoe, 2011).

As with some of the other care groups discussed in Part 2 of the book, people with reduced intellectual capacity may experience forms of discrimination and stigma. This excerpt from Patient Opinion illustrates how stigma is applied.

Patient (and family) story 7.1

We arrived at ******** city hospital Opthomology depart with our foster child who has Down's syndrome. He had been referred to the hospital by the optician. We were very disappointed with the doctor who treated. The doctor said that our foster child had been diagnosed with eye problems in September 2012 but there was nothing he could do as he had a disability and this was probably why he was struggling at school.

I cannot believe that in this day and age a professional could have such an attitude towards someone with a disability. We do not know whether our foster child is having more difficulties with learning because of his sight and would have thought that despite his disability options would be explored as to what could be done. We were basically told that nothing could be done as he has a disability. (www.patientopinion.org.uk/, 2015)

The term covers a range of disabilities. The communication needs of some individuals may be such that the use of pre-verbal/pre-intentional communication or early gestures (which include touch, eye contact, smiling, etc.) might be the most appropriate form of communication.

This is not in any sense 'baby talk', but simply a way of acknowledging the stage of language development in that individual and the need for this to be considered when developing their communicative potential. Other people may be able to sustain verbal communication relatively successfully.

According to Martin, O'Connor-Fenelon and Lyons (2012a), the most consistent and frequently identified aspect of communication with people who have an intellectual disability is familiarity and really knowing the person. Familiarity refers to the nurse knowing not only the person's communication methods, but also their background, family situation, physical health, psychological and behavioural health and patterns, likes/dislikes, etc. – in fact, every aspect of their life. In keeping with a person-centred philosophy and associated principles, this individualised knowledge and familiarity lie at the centre not only of the communication exchange but also of the nurse–service user relationship; indeed, it is the very essence of both and can be utilised to maximise the probability of communication being successful.

Certain themes are evident within this concept of familiarity, including emotional conflict, the need to listen for tone and pitch of verbal aspects of communication and also to observe non-verbal communication alongside the way in which the individual conveys messages (Martin et al., 2012b). When a nurse first meets someone with an intellectual disability, they may find communication with them difficult as they do not have this knowledge of them as a person and, at this point in the nurse–patient relationship, it is important to draw on the knowledge of others who have this familiarity. However, as the knowledge of the person builds up, the nurse sees their personal characteristics and baseline behaviours and can then use these to inform future communication.

Total Communication (TC) is an approach developed to create a successful and equal communication between people with different language perception and/or production (Pardoe, 2011). It is concerned with exploring all aspects of communication to discover what is best for the individual and therefore depends on a nurse's familiarity with them. TC asks nurses to stop and think before they assume that their preferred method of communication is also shared by the person they are interacting with. All forms of communication have value in TC, and different forms may be appropriate in different situations and for specific people. Rather than imposing their own preferred techniques and maintaining them despite their inadequacies with an individual with intellectual disabilities, TC requires nurses to be innovative and creative, and to look at all the alternative ways in which messages can be sent and received. The nurse can then employ the most effective approach for that specific individual rather than one which is controlling and disempowering (Pardoe, 2011).

CRITICAL THINKING EXERCISE 7.1
REDUCED CAPACITY TO COMMUNICATE

Think of a time when your normally preferred method of communication became difficult or even impossible – maybe because of illness or environment. What did you do? What other forms of communication did you employ to ensure your interactions were effective?

Visit the Values Exchange website at http://sagecomms.vxcommunity.com to develop your critical thinking skills and debate your thoughts and decisions.

It has already been noted that some people with intellectual disabilities have such extreme communication needs that comprehension of any spoken word is difficult because they have not yet begun (or had opportunities) to develop the foundation skills of communication. Attempting to facilitate understanding through spoken words is likely to be unsuccessful and alternative approaches will need to be found in order to enable clients to engage with their world and with the nurses themselves. Other individuals may be able to receive some fairly complex ideas through the spoken word, but will not necessarily be able to decode some of the additional components that accompany such conversations, such as the use of metaphor or sarcasm. It is easy to over-estimate a person's understanding or receptive language skills as they may be able to disguise their limitations in a variety of ways. These include using non-verbal cues and familiarity with routine to make sense of events without necessarily understanding the words spoken at the time – for example, the arrival of a tea trolley in a room may initiate a response of 'Cup of tea, please' without a full understanding of the words spoken by the healthcare professional pushing the trolley.

If nurses wish to enhance their ability to make themselves understood more effectively, it is important to know those people with intellectual disabilities well and use other strategies alongside verbal means to strengthen what needs to be communicated. With regard to verbal aspects of communication, TC would suggest considering the following areas:

- using short, straightforward sentences
- maintaining consistent use of vocabulary
- emphasising important words
- slowing speech, whilst maintaining its rhythm
- avoiding abstract concepts and ideas.

When considering an individual's expressive ability, it is important to recognise that they may have developed a range of 'stock' phrases (for example, 'Good afternoon, is it time for tea?' or 'I'm going out, I am'), which may be clearly articulated but are used in a wide variety of situations, in many of which these phrases are not appropriate. They are being used for a purpose other than that which the actual content of the message might be considered to convey. It is therefore also important not to over-estimate someone's expressive ability simply on the basis of the language they use. There may be other difficulties associated with expression which relate to articulation and fluency due to, for example, physical issues, stammering, and making expressive language more difficult to deliver and receive (Pardoe, 2011).

TC suggests the following strategies to foster expressive communication:

- Encourage people to use the form of communication that works for them.
- Always be prepared to give time to the speaker.
- Accept their communication without judgement.
- Make judicious use of questioning.
- Use visual aids.

However, it is often necessary to supplement verbal communication with some other strategy such as Augmentative and Alternative Communication (AAC). Particularly when verbal communication is not the preferred mode of interaction or when verbal communication is difficult to understand, people with intellectual disability can be offered a strategy which either augments their existing skills or provides an effective alternative (Cockerill et al., 2013). There are two types of AAC – unaided systems which require no external devices and include manual signs and gestures, and aided strategies which require external assistance in the form of picture cards, electronic speech devices or alphabet boards (Trembath et al., 2014).

Some examples of AAC include Intensive Interaction, signing systems and Signalong. Intensive Interaction is based on a model of caregiver–infant interaction and works by focusing on the quality of everyday interactions. It is a method of engagement which tries to respond to what the individual brings to an interaction, allowing them to take the lead and share fully in the give-and-take that characterises most episodes of effective communication, which is both valuing and empowering. Signing systems are often used in addition to, or in conjunction with, the spoken word to support efforts to articulate even if these are indistinct. An example of this is the Makaton system which involves the use of speech, symbols and signs derived from British Sign Language (BSL). Signalong is another sign-supporting system based on BSL which empowers children and adults with impaired communication related to intellectual disabilities to understand and express their needs, choices and desires by providing a vocabulary for both life and learning (Pardoe, 2011).

Communicating with people who have dementia

AAC is applicable not only in the care of those with intellectual disabilities, but also for people with dementia. Dementia refers to a group of conditions which result in a decline in mental ability affecting memory, thinking, problem solving, concentration and perception (Mental Health Foundation, 2009). One such condition is Alzheimer's Disease in which dense bundles of abnormal fibres are found in the cytoplasm of neurones whose axons and dendrites may also show signs of alteration (senile plaques) (Jootun and McGhee, 2011). Other forms of dementia include vascular dementia in which there are changes in the cerebral blood vessel, dementia with Lewy bodies (abnormal clumps of protein in the central cortex) and mixed dementia.

Whatever the form of dementia, as the definition above suggests, the condition will usually affect memory and orientation to time, place and person. The gradual decrease in cognitive ability associated with the condition means that the ability to think and communicate progressively declines and the individual finds it increasingly difficult to process new information (Veselinova, 2014). An early sign that an individual's ability to communicate is being compromised by dementia is that they cannot find the words to express what they want to say, particularly in regard to the names of objects (Jootun and McGhee, 2011). They may substitute an incorrect word, or may not find any word at all.

Over time, people with dementia may lose the ability to understand what is being said to them and struggle with verbal expression. As a consequence, they may participate less in social situations, due to losing the capacity to understand interactions. This can lead to feelings of isolation and frustration and may result in the individual withdrawing from society and risking additional health problems such as anxiety and depression.

Veselinova (2014) notes how dementia also affects the ability to present rational ideas. Memory impairment can make verbal language more difficult, both in speaking and understanding.

Wang et al. (2013) found that some nurses who had less education in the effects of dementia, had difficulty in understanding and communicating with their patients. Their attempts to persuade patients to exhibit 'normal' behaviour simply served to reinforce confusion and disorientation.

Nursing story 7.1: (Mis)interpretations of behaviour

I don't understand what he means, don't know what he needs. He makes some noise but I cannot help him. (Alzheimer's type, end stage; nurse D)

He says he has a stomachache every day! After a while, he says he has no pain at all and another area hurts! We are confused! (Alzheimer's type, late stage; nurse F)

Sometimes I wonder what are the meanings of their postures or behavior? (nurse I); Sometimes I said to myself 'Oh, my goodness, what does this mean!' I really have no idea what they tried to express their needs. (nurse J)

No matter what I said to him, he wouldn't stop his behavior, he just wondered around and continuously made noise. (Alzheimer's type, end stage; nurse F)

(Wang et al., 2013, p. 102)

 Visit the Values Exchange website at http://sagecomms.vxcommunity.com for a broader discussion on this Nursing story.

As Wang et al. (2013) noted, the nurses tried to reinforce reality and to reason with people who had lost the ability to reason. This simply made the situation more difficult for all concerned.

Whilst every person with dementia is unique and their behaviour cannot be attributed solely to the condition, there is no doubt that the progressive decline in their ability to communicate does pose a challenge to nurses seeking to provide high quality care. The person-centred approach to care and communication stresses the need to acknowledge the uniqueness and individuality of every person when assessing their ability to communicate, making it clear that the responsibility to facilitate communication with someone with dementia lies with the nurse.

People with dementia and their families can describe widely variable experiences of care, as demonstrated below in Patient story 7.1 with a tale from a cognitive impairment and dementia centre.

Patient (and family) story 7.1

The care my Mother has received from Dr *****-**** and ***** at St ********** has been exemplary.

Both parties have shown a very clear and compassionate understanding of my Mother's condition and we will be forever grateful for their endless patience and support.

***** has been marvellous in following up at every stage. An outstanding service, thank you both.'

But also

A relative with cognitive impairment admitted with acute physical health care symptoms was treated with no dignity, zero respect, main focus was his mental state and how he was draining resources due to requiring special obs

Informed that ward ** had 16 patients and not enough staff, relying on agency staff that did not know the patients

Despite the cognitive impairment and the hospital advertising dementia initiatives my grandfather was moved 5 times in 5 days

When asked for treatment plan and diagnosis told do not know

Daily informed of different information all conflicting ranging from a call to say he's medically fit to 6 hours later he's being moved again to a rehab ward for 3 weeks

Asked how they are treating the infection told lorazepam

Attempts to speak to senior management failed

Attempts to speak to Matron failed

Now hoping bed manager promise to call back will happen but so far proving not to live in hope

Standard of care not good enough

No evidence to suggest compassionate care never mind advocating independence and MDT working that holds the patient and carer at the centre.

(www.patientopinion.org.uk/, 2016)

Whereas the first experience in Patient story 7.1 was positive, the second was negative.
The following list illustrates the verbal language difficulties for people with dementia:

- choosing an incorrect word to express feelings
- only being able to find single words to express complex feelings
- talking fluently but words do not appear to make sense
- creating new words where meaning is not clear
- choosing words that are similar in meaning or sound like the intended word, but are not quite accurate
- repeating sounds and words that others say, but without understanding
- losing the ability to start or follow a conversation
- misunderstanding communication
- using challenging or demanding language, including swearing.

Engaging with people who have dementia may be mutually satisfying or frustrating when a nurse encounters difficulties. It is therefore important to develop specific strategies to facilitate effective communication with these individuals.

The following list identifies a range of skills from the nurse's everyday 'toolkit' which can be used to promote effective communication with a person who has dementia:

- Approach the person from the front.
- Make sure to face the person when speaking to them.
- Give the person some cues – e.g. a touch of the arm/hand – or use their name before starting an interaction.
- Ensure the environment is quiet and free from distractions.

- Use simple language and speak slowly.
- Use short and simple sentences.
- Speak to the person as an adult.
- Do not speak in the person's presence as if they were not there.
- Give the person time to complete their thoughts and to struggle with words.
- Avoid being too quick to guess what the person is trying to express.
- Repeat sentences in a neutral tone.
- Encourage the individual to write down the word they are trying to express and read it aloud.
- Use appropriate facial expressions even though it may feel a bit exaggerated.
- Do not correct the person if they make mistakes.
- Do not pressure the person to respond.
- Encourage the person to use any mode of communication with which they feel comfortable.
- Use touch to aid concentration, to establish another means of communication and to offer reassurance/encouragement.
- Avoid contradicting and arguing with the person. (Alzheimer's Society, 2010)

Many of these skills will sound familiar as they are also considered valuable in Total Communication, as discussed earlier in this chapter. However, regardless of how good the communication toolkit and skills of nurses, they are not necessarily sufficient to ensure high quality communication unless there is greater attention paid to the qualitative characteristics of the relationship that nurses develop with people who have dementia (McEvoy and Plant, 2014). Every individual is a relational being and the empathic interactions that they have with others have significant effects on both their sense of self and how they feel about the world. Empathic responses communicate an appreciation of what other people are experiencing and can help to build feelings of connection, mutuality and trust. Empathy can be defined as understanding another person's frame of mind and behaviour by putting oneself in their place (Stueber, 2012). Key aspects of empathy include tuning in to the emotional experiences of others, drawing inferences about their mental state and responding with professional concern (McEvoy and Plant, 2014).

Empathic curiosity is a metacommunicative position which a nurse can adopt when trying to focus their attention on the personal experiences of someone with dementia, as that person is experiencing them. Metacommunication relates to the tone that is communicated, rather than what is actually said or done. The underlying tone may resonate at an emotional level and reflect the feelings of an individual more powerfully than any words the nurse may use (McEvoy and Plant, 2014). Empathic curiosity can help to foster greater engagement and insight by opening up communication spaces in which people can share their self-awareness and life experiences.

It is facilitated by empathic listening which involves paying close attention to the minute particulars that occur during conversations. When communicating with someone who has dementia, this will involve identifying cues, including non-verbal disruptions in the flow of conversation, metaphorical clues that may signal emotional concerns or needs, and asking short, non-intrusive questions that open up space for the individual to talk about their current experience. Adopting a curious attitude helps to direct attention towards the reasons behind a person's behaviour, their specific concerns and the personal values that are meaningful to them.

The pace and control of the conversation is another aspect of communication which is important when interacting with someone who has dementia, enabling them to have sufficient time to think, find their words (again, also aspects of TC) and share the responsibility for sustaining conversation in a collaborative way that allows them to regain some control over the interaction whilst assimilating information. If people with dementia are not given the space and time they need to think things through and identify the words they want to say, they may not be able to reach their full communicative potential. Facilitating this involvement in conversation promotes a feeling of subjective wellbeing in the person with dementia, which will, in turn, encourage them to become involved in future interactions.

AAC was identified as being an important aspect of communication with people with intellectual disabilities and it also has a role to play with those with dementia. Talking Mats can be used by many, but not all, people with intellectual disabilities (Murphy and Cameron, 2008) and those with dementia, being of particular value for those in the early or middle stages of the condition. Talking Mats are a low-technology communication framework which use a simple system of picture symbols, placed on a textured mat, that allow people to indicate their feelings about various options within a topic by placing the relevant image below a visual scale. They are accessible, inexpensive and can be used in any care setting to enhance the communicative ability of people with dementia.

Murphy and Oliver (2013) suggest that Talking Mats improve the length of time that a person with early-stage dementia maintains concentration in an interaction as well as their ability to keep on track during the interaction, both of which increase the extent to which their communication partners understand their views. In addition, Talking Mats help to clarify the thoughts of someone with dementia and enable them to express their views. This then provides a means through which these individuals can convey their thoughts to both family carers and nurses, facilitating the achievement of joint decisions and ensuring that the voice of the person with dementia is heard. Family carers of people with dementia acknowledge the value of Talking Mats in encouraging and maintaining communication and allowing them to have a better understanding of their family member.

For nurses caring for people with dementia, as well as for the individual themselves and their family, living well with dementia involves a complex balancing act as they negotiate a way through changing needs and preferences in everyday life as well as choices regarding current and future management of their care. Talking Mats provide a framework whereby the needs and values of the person and their family can be expressed and then incorporated into ongoing plans and packages of care. By facilitating conversations of this nature, it may be possible for a nurse to identify the individual's and family's strengths and abilities, correct misconceptions about abilities and preferences, alleviate anxiety on behalf of both the person with dementia and their carers, and allow the expression of concerns in a safe and non-confrontational way (Murphy and Oliver, 2013).

Critical debate 7.1

Do we do enough to educate in communicating with people with cognitive deficits?

Conclusion

Communication skills present in the toolkit of every nurse can be employed in interactions with people who have diminished intellectual capacity, but they are often not enough. This chapter has explored how these so-called 'basic' skills can be adapted for use with this particular client group, and it has become apparent that skills important in Total Communication with people with intellectual disability can also play a role in interactions with those with dementia. However, additional strategies are often also required, of which there are many.

Only a few have been addressed, but the importance of Augmentative and Alternative Communication in both intellectual disability and the care of those with dementia has been highlighted along with the value of nurses adopting an empathic curiosity.

References

Alzheimer's Society (2010) *Advice for Nurses and other Healthcare Professionals.* Available at: www.alzheimers.org.uk/site/scripts/documents_info.php?documentID=1211&pageNumber=2 (accessed 10 January 16).

Cockerill, H., Elbourne, D., Allen, E., Scrutton, D., Will, E., McNee, A., et al. (2013) 'Speech communication and the use of augmentative communication in young people with cerebral palsy: the SH&PE population study', *Child: Care, Health and Development*, 40(2): 149–57.

Jootun, D. and McGhee, G. (2011) 'Effective communication with people who have dementia', *Nursing Standard*, 25(25): 40–6.

Martin, A.-M., O'Connor-Fenelon, M. and Lyons, R. (2012a) 'Non-verbal communication between registered nurses' intellectual disability and people with an intellectual disability: an exploratory study of the nurse's experiences – part 1', *Journal of Intellectual Disabilities*, 16(1): 61–75.

Martin, A.-M., O'Connor-Fenelon, M. and Lyons, R. (2012b) 'Non-verbal communication between registered nurses' intellectual disability and people with an intellectual disability: an exploratory study of the nurse's experiences – part 2', *Journal of Intellectual Disabilities*, 16(2): 97–108.

McEvoy, P. and Plant, R. (2014) 'Dementia care: using empathic curiosity to establish the common ground that is necessary for meaningful communication', *Journal of Psychiatric and Mental Health Nursing*, 21(6): 477–82.

Mental Health Foundation (2009) *Dementia.* Available from www.mentalhealth.org.uk/a-to-z/d/dementia(accessed 27/1/16).

Morris, G. and Morris, J. (2010) *The Dementia Care Workbook.* Maidenhead: Open University Press.

Murphy, J. and Cameron, L. (2008) 'The effectiveness of Talking Mats with people with intellectual disability', *British Journal of Learning Disabilities*, 36(4): 232–41.

Murphy, J. and Oliver, T. (2013) 'The use of Talking Mats to support people with dementia and their carers to make decisions together', *Health and Social Care in the Community*, 21(2): 171–80.

Pardoe, R. (2011) 'Promoting effective communication', in E. Broussine and K. Scarborough (eds), *Supporting People with Learning Disabilities in Health and Social Care*. London: Sage.

Stueber, K.R. (2012) 'Varieties of empathy, neuroscience and the narrativist challenge to the contemporary theory of mind debate', *Emotion Review*, 4(1): 55–63.

Trembath, D., Iaconon, T., Lyon, K., West, D. and Johnson, H. (2014) 'Augmentative and alternative communication supports for adults with autism spectrum disorders', *Autism*, 18(8): 891–902.

Veselinova, C. (2014) 'Influencing communication and interaction in dementia', *Nursing and Residential Care*, 16(3): 162–6.

Wang, J., Hsieh, P. and Wang, J. (2013) 'Long-term care nurses' communication difficulties with people living with dementia in Taiwan', *Asian Nursing Research*, 7: 99–103.

Useful websites

Dementia Friends: An Alzeimer's Society Initiative home page – www.dementiafriends.org.uk
Headway: The Brain Injury Association home page – www.headway.org.uk
Mencap: The Voice of Learning Disability home page – www.mencap.org.uk/
Mental Health Foundation on dementia – www.mentalhealth.org.uk/tags/dementia

 To access further resources related to this chapter, visit the Values Exchange website at http://sagecomms.vxcommunity.com

8

Communicating with Children, Young People and Families

Jean Shapcott

• • • • • • • • • • • Learning Objectives • • • • • • • • • • • •

By the end of this chapter, you will have developed an understanding of:

- communicating within the context of the family
- how development affects communication
- stereotyping young people.

Don't forget to visit the Values Exchange website at http://sagecomms.vxcommunity.com for extra practice and revision activities.

• •

Introduction

As identified in earlier chapters, of all the healthcare professionals, the nurse is the one who will spend the most time with children, young people and their families in healthcare settings. As a result, they are the ones who regularly encounter children who are frightened and distressed by their illness and its implications, particularly if these include a sudden and unexpected change in their situation such as hospitalisation. An admission to hospital can result in increased anxiety and behavioural regression, both of which can have an impact on a child's ability to communicate effectively. However, even when illness and hospitalisation make reciprocation difficult, it is essential that nurses focus their communication on children and young people. The *United Nations Convention on the Rights of the Child* (UNCRC) (1989) includes the need to take into consideration the views not only of parents, but also those of children and young people themselves, emphasising the importance of listening to children and considering their views as well as taking account of parents' responsibility to act in the best interest of their child.

Child- and family-centred care is both a core element and a fundamental principle in nursing children. The family is recognised as a constant in the life of most children (Lambert, 2012) and it is therefore important to remember that parents should normally be involved in all aspects of their child's care, one of the few exceptions to this rule being where there might be safeguarding concerns regarding a family member. The nurse must also acknowledge that, depending on their age and stage of development, the child or young person should be involved in any decisions made regarding them and their care. Effective communication is therefore a vital part of child- and family-centred care and this is what will be explored in this chapter.

Defining child- and family-centred care

For Kuo et al., family-centred care (FCC) is defined as 'a partnership approach to health care decision-making between the family and health care provider. FCC is considered the standard of paediatric health care by many clinical practices, hospitals, and health care groups' (2012, p. 297). However, they note that, in practice, this concept remains testing for both practitioners and families.

Communication with children, young people and their families can be both challenging and rewarding, often at the same time. The Nursing and Midwifery Council (2015) recognises the importance of nurses being able to establish and maintain dynamic, reciprocal and therapeutic relationships not only with their young patients, but also with members of the family and others who children and young people perceive as significant in their lives. This can also prove challenging, particularly, for example, in situations where parents believe they are protecting their child by withholding specific information from them, whilst the child or young person themselves may be acutely aware that there is something wrong in the interactions they are having with their parents or the nurse. When faced with a scenario of this nature, it might seem easier for the nurse to withdraw and simply follow the lead of the parents, but this will simply serve to widen the web of deceit and reduce the child's or young person's willingness to trust nursing staff. Knowing how to communicate effectively with children, young people and families will provide nurses with a toolkit from which to draw in any situation.

CRITICAL THINKING EXERCISE 8.1
REFLECTION ON CHILDHOOD

Spend five minutes writing down your memories of being a child. What issues and themes were significant for you at that time in your life? What did it feel like to move into being an adolescent/ young person? Did those themes and issues change?

Communicating within the context of the family

It is already clear that, in the context of caring for children and young people, communication is not a simple two-way process. Nurses are under an obligation to encourage the active participation of both children/young people and parents in decision making and care. Their ability to do this is dependent on the ability to manage the dynamics of a three-way dialogical relationship between themselves, the child or young person and their parents in the context of busy healthcare settings or in their own home (Lambert, 2012).

The triad of communication

Caring for children involves nurses in three-way, triadic interactions between themselves, the child or young person and their parent(s). It is important to recognise that some children do want to be represented by their parents, maybe because they feel too ill to do it themselves, they want to limit their own exposure to potentially worrying information or they may simply be unable to understand what the nurse is trying to communicate to them. Consequently, they assume the passive bystander position on the continuum, by choice, as they observe the dyadic (two-way) interaction between their parent and the nurse (Callery and Milnes, 2012), whilst remaining part of the triadic relationship.

With the involvement of a third party, namely the parent or other family member, the dynamics of any interaction become increasingly complex. Parents often assume an intermediary role between the nurse and their child (Lambert, 2012), which may either support effective communication or inhibit it. Supportive roles assumed by the parent include acting as a communication buffer for their child by indicating when the interaction needs to end, answering difficult questions for them, empowering their child to participate in the interaction and discussion, and enhancing their memory of events and understanding of information (Gibson et al., 2010; Van Staa, 2011). However, whilst children value these supportive roles, they also also indicate their dissatisfaction at some of the ways in which they feel parents inhibit their attempts to participate by answering questions on their behalf, insisting that they stay quiet, reprimanding them for interrupting discussions, withholding information or filtering the information they want their child to hear and not supporting attempts to get the information the child believes they need (Coyne and Gallagher, 2011; Van Staa, 2011).

Often considered to be nothing more than multi-party talk in which children are passive bystanders, it is important for any nurse involved in the care of children to acknowledge that parents may sometimes be the ones on the sidelines (Callery and Milnes, 2012). This is most likely to occur when the child is an expert in their own condition or in the care of an older child or young person who, by virtue of their age and stage of development, is more able to articulate needs or preferences and be an active participant in interactions.

As well as the potential for co-operation within the triadic relationship, there is also the risk of conflict. This may occur within the dyads of child/parent, nurse/parent or nurse/child, or the wider triad, and adds to the complexity of this communication pattern, whilst having implications for the therapeutic potential of the triadic relationship. Therapeutic relationships require the nurse to relate closely to the experience of children/young people and their families and the way in which they interpret events, challenges and needs, in order that they might feel they have been heard and understood (Roberts et al., 2015). Nurses must therefore show their trustworthiness through demonstrating professional attributes within the triadic interactions. Patient story 8.1 is an example of the family reaction when this happens.

Patient (family) story 8.1: 'Amazing care'

My son fractured his arm playing football. From the friendly staff in a very busy A&E to the amazing staff in the children's ward and the reassuring and friendly theatre staff the experience was as good as these things can be.

We were fully informed at all times and all the staff in the children's ward did an excellent job in looking after my son and his mum.

The follow up care and friendly staff at the fracture clinic have continued the positive experience. In a busy and demanding environment the staff go above and beyond to provide fantastic care. (www.patientopinion.org.uk/, 2016)

In Student story 8.1, a student nurse blogger describes how she enjoys interaction with families and children.

Student story 8.1

I really enjoy interacting with children and their parents and helping to put them at ease in difficult and scary situations. One of my favourite things about my job is being able to explain what will be happening to patients and their parents and see how they are reassured and then just able to focus on getting better and going home. (student. blogs.anglia.ac.uk/tag/child-nursing/)

Communicating with children and young people

Young children rely on adults to make decisions on their behalf because they lack the necessary understanding of their condition and associated treatment. However, with maturity comes increasing understanding and autonomy and consequently an enhanced ability to be involved in care decisions. Nurses must therefore monitor relationships with children and young people, recognising the vulnerability of the child, whilst addressing all aspects of their physical and emotional wellbeing. Children and young people are very clear about what they want from nurses with regard to communication and, if nurses are to address these factors, they need a sound knowledge of the impact that the age of the child and their stage of development has on communication.

What children and young people say they want

Children and young people need information to be communicated to them in a format which they can access and understand, in order to be able to know what to expect in relation to their condition, forthcoming procedures, medication and the length of time they may need to stay in hospital. Many children and young people believe they have a right to be involved in discussions and decisions about their care because it involves them directly and, of course, they are the people experiencing the condition or healthcare situation. Therefore, they want to participate in communication exchanges and have their viewpoints or concerns taken seriously.

However, many children report that they experience difficulties achieving this participation, indicating that one of the main factors preventing this is the communication style and behaviour of healthcare professionals (Coyne and Gallagher, 2011). Children say that nurses tend to 'do things' to them with only a very brief explanation, or even no explanation at all. Many indicate that they feel unable to ask questions or volunteer information because nurses appear too rushed and busy during the interactions they have with them. Children also feel that nurses seem to direct information at parents, relegating children to non-participant observer status and forcing them to rely on parents to advocate on their behalf (Coyne and Gallagher, 2011).

Lambert, Glacken and McCarron (2011) suggest that children and young people occupy a position on a 'visible-ness' communication continuum which moves from being passive bystanders, as described above, to becoming active participants in interactions, according to the child's exclusion or inclusion in the communication process and the extent to which their communication needs are met. According to Lambert (2012), a child's or young person's position on this continuum is influenced by perceptions of children, including the perception of children as immature, incompetent and dependent versus an opposing view that children can become mature, competent and independent. These opposing views are reflective of an overarching tension between the protection of children and their participation in all aspects of care, which presents yet another challenge to nurses wishing to communicate effectively with children. As a consequence of the positions assumed by children and young people on this continuum and their expressed difficulties in communication, their expressed preferences are often ignored, which then further undermines their participation in interactions and may result in increased trauma due to their lack of understanding of procedures and nursing interventions.

How development affects communication

No two children, even identical twins, are the same in the way they develop and communicate. Most children use recognisable words during their second year and are likely to know at least 50 words and combine them in short phrases by the age of 2 years. Once a child's vocabulary reaches about 200 words, the rate of word learning increases dramatically and the ability to apply grammatical rules begins. During early childhood (3–5 years), sentence patterns become increasingly complex and vocabulary diversifies to include relational terms that express notions of size, location, quantity and time. From this point onwards, children learn to use language more effectively and efficiently. They learn how to create and maintain larger language units, such as conversation or narrative, until eventually achieving a full vocabulary as well as conversational ability as an adolescent (Johnson, 2005).

However, there are a range of factors that might result in children not developing some aspects of language. These include physical factors such as hearing impairment, a cleft lip or palate that has not been fully repaired or the enlarged tongue associated with Down's syndrome. The verbal environment also influences a child's development of language. Children who grow up in a family characterised by an extensive vocabulary and well-structured language are likely to emulate this in their own development, whilst those from families where language use is limited may lag behind (Hart and Risley, 1995). Poor language development may be part of a wider issue such as global developmental delay. It is clear that nurses caring for children and young people must understand that age is not the only factor to determine the language and communicative ability of a child and should always recognise their individuality in any interactions.

There are some useful guidelines for communicating with children. These include using age-appropriate language so as to ensure that young children understand what is being said, whilst ensuring that older children and adolescents do not feel patronised. When communicating with younger children, it is really important to get down to their level since this reduces (to some extent) the perceived power difference between children and adults.

The cry of an infant is a powerful signal used in order to communicate and receive a timely response. It is therefore important to respond to a crying infant in a timely fashion since, if left to cry, they miss out on an important opportunity for learning to trust those caring for them. Older infants, particularly those over eight months of age, develop stranger anxiety so it is important to spend time with them and their parents to enable the infant to get to know the nurses caring for them. Infants are able to engage in play and, from a young age, can focus on facial expression. They love the sound of the human voice, particularly when a calm and soothing tone is employed. Older infants will raise their arms, indicating that they wish to be lifted up, play peek-a-boo and break eye contact when they have had enough stimulation or playtime. It is therefore clear that non-verbal cues are evident in children from a very early age.

Toddlers are usually described using two characteristic methods of communication – they constantly use the word 'why?' and they exhibit tantrums associated with the 'terrible two's'. However, in healthcare settings they are often fearful and quickly resistant, so it is important to approach them carefully and use the calm, soothing tone preferred by infants. Toddlers need to respond to nurses in their own time, so, whenever possible, they should be allowed to do so. It is also important to ask parents what words the toddler uses for specific things and actions in order to facilitate understanding.

Children aged 3–5 years are full of curiosity and the desire to explore and create. This can be used to the nurse's advantage in communication since children of this age are keen to establish good relationships with adults and peers, and are learning to reason and solve problems as they become more independent. They enjoy stories, rhymes and music, all of which can be used as a medium for communication. It is important that nurses are clear and honest, using simple, interconnected terms since, despite their growing vocabulary, the ability to understand complex sentences should not be taken for granted. When ill, children in this age group experience a vast array of feelings, many of which may be new and uncomfortable. Nurses can use the language of feelings, encouraging them to draw as well as talk about their feelings and fears, what they do and do not like and any choices they may have. The key to effective communication with very young children is to be clear, but light-hearted.

School-age children (5–11 years) have enhanced verbal skills and are therefore better able to express their feelings. Third-party stories can be used to elicit information from them, for example 'how might you...?', 'what if that were you...?', as it provides a less direct approach, allowing children to voice their concerns and/or ask questions that they might not otherwise be able to ask.

A contemporary understanding of adolescence appears to be rooted in the notion of transition (Coleman, 2011), as the young person moves from being a child to becoming an adult. Social inconsistencies and variations in accepted practice with regard to the legal age at which activities may be undertaken make it difficult to define the roles and responsibilities of young people receiving care. A key concept for nurses communicating with young people and involving them in decision making is that of Gillick competence (*Gillick v West*

Norfolk and Wisbech Area Health Authority, 1986), and nurses must ensure that this is assessed and acknowledged whenever it is applicable.

CRITICAL THINKING EXERCISE 8.2
GILLICK COMPETENCE

- What is Gillick competence?
- Consider how healthcare professionals might assess a young person's Gillick competence?
- Does whether a young person is Gillick competent change the way in which nurses communicate with them?

Visit the Values Exchange website at http://sagecomms.vxcommunity.com to develop your critical thinking skills and debate your thoughts and decisions.

Stereotyping young people

Young people are often stereotyped in UK society. These assumptions about adolescents as a group, rather than as individuals, have the potential to remove the uniqueness and personal characteristics of a young person by replacing them with a set of limited, predictable and generalised qualities that are ascribed to every member of the group. Stereotypes can very easily become destructive and limit nurses' capacity to communicate with young people in an unbiased, non-judgemental manner, since they may lead to prejudice, conflict and hostility.

CRITICAL THINKING EXERCISE 8.3
THINKING ABOUT YOUNG PEOPLE

- How do you view adolescents/teenagers/young people?
- What is the origin of these views?
- Have you any stereotypes regarding this age group?
- How are you going to minimise the impact of these stereotypes in your communication?

Visit the Values Exchange website at http://sagecomms.vxcommunity.com to develop your critical thinking skills and debate your thoughts and decisions.

Young people may be receptive or hostile to healthcare. They may actively seek parental involvement in decision making and care or prefer them to be excluded and may themselves be carers for a family member (McAndrew et al., 2012). They expect a range of attributes and skills from nurses including those related to communication, namely being available and accepting, informed and informative, empathic and able to ensure privacy and dignity within the healthcare environment (Robinson, 2010). However, some factors can hinder nurses' communication with young people. These include a negative attitude towards this age group and focusing on parents or the medical condition itself, rather than on the impact it may be having on everyday life, education or emotional wellbeing (Fallon, 2012).

One of the most complex tasks for nurses communicating with young people is negotiation of their confidentiality, whilst maintaining the confidence of their parent(s). Young people report experiencing difficulty being afforded some time to discuss issues privately, particularly those of a sensitive nature, and many do not even get asked if they want to be seen alone (Mappa et al., 2010). Nurses cite the need to include the parent as part of the team, time constraints and perceptions that it is unnecessary as reasons for this. Whilst continuing to recognise the individuality of each young person and the need to work within legal frameworks, it is important for nurses to negotiate some of these complex issues, balancing parental involvement with a young person's need for privacy and acknowledging that the priorities of the different parties may differ.

Using play and technology in communication

Play is an integral part of a child's life, having a major role in development and providing a means through which children can explore and express emotions. Behind the apparent simplicity of play lies a complexity in which ideas, understanding, exploration and communication are pursued (Binns and Hicks, 2012).

Play can be used to address the negative consequences of healthcare, for example hospitalisation, through reducing stress, providing an outlet for anxiety and offering a diversion from unpleasant procedures and treatments. Using play strategies such as dressing up, music, drawing, as well as messy or water play, can provide effective preparation for procedures and reduce the trauma that may result. Play as a distraction aims to take a child's mind off a procedure by concentrating on something else, for example bubbles blown by a nurse, or a puppet.

Recent advantages in technology have resulted in communication interventions that offer possibilities for distraction as well as education about conditions and healthcare. These include use of the Internet, virtual reality and online support groups. Social media provide a multitude of opportunities for communication, particularly when coupled with rapidly developing mobile technology, as young people can maintain easy communication with peers even during hospitalisation which might otherwise destabilise these important relationships (Fallon, 2012). Young people are also avid users of texting and multimedia through these mobile devices and these media can be used to communicate reminders of appointments or medication; the growing importance of these technologies to communication should not be underestimated (Binns and Hicks, 2012).

With the Internet now being the primary source of healthcare information for many young people, it is important that nurses are aware of the potential risks of this environment. These include unintentional disclosure of personal information, bullying and harassment and the targeting of users by predators. Whilst every effort can be made to ensure that young people can access their social media, Internet safety must be maintained in healthcare environments.

Amongst the complexity inherent in communication with children, young people and families, tools such as the Simple Skills Secret (Jack et al., 2013) can be utilised to communicate effectively with children and parents. Child and family centredness can be enhanced by the use of open questions focused on matters of importance to individuals and the whole family linked to a verbal or non-verbal cue, and by encouraging children, young people and families to seek their own solutions to problems, no matter how complex, individually or collectively, rather than requiring nurses to engage in a long, in-depth conversation or discussion for which they feel unprepared or unskilled. Given the complexity of communication with children, young people and parents, it is important that nurses utilise any such tools or other supportive measures to ensure the message is clearly transmitted and effectively understood.

Critical debate 8.1

Are young people and adolescents demonised by society? Discuss.

Conclusion

This chapter has explored communication with children, young people and families at the earlier stages of the lifespan. As with other chapters in this book, we stress that good communication is about recognising the context of the care group and about monitoring ourselves. There are certain specific skills for communicating with children and young people but much of this skill capacity centres on an awareness of the developmental stage of the child or young person. Play, technology and the child's level of competence may be unique to childhood, but, as with all groups across the lifespan, the willingness of the nurse to engage in communication appropriate to the context is of utmost importance.

References

Binns, F. and Hicks, P. (2012) 'Using play and technology to communicate with children and young people', in V. Lambert, T. Long and D. Kelleher (eds), *Communication Skills for Children's Nurses*. Maidenhead: McGraw-Hill.

Callery, P. and Milnes, L. (2012) 'Communication between nurses, children and their parents in asthma review consultations', *Journal of Clinical Nursing*, 21(11–12): 1641–50.

Coleman, J. (2011) *Adolescence*, 4th edn. Hove: Routledge.

Coyne, I. and Gallagher, P. (2011) 'Participation in communication and decision-making: children and young people's experiences in a hospital setting', *Journal of Clinical Nursing*, 20(15–16): 2334–43.

Fallon, D. (2012) 'Communicating with young people', in V. Lambert, T. Long and D. Kelleher (eds), *Communication Skills for Children's Nurses*. Maidenhead: McGraw-Hill.

Gibson, F., Aldiss, S., Horstman, M., Kumpunen, S. and Richardson, A. (2010) 'Children and young people's experiences of cancer care: a qualitative research study using participatory methods', *International Journal of Nursing Studies*, 47(11): 1397–1407.

Gillick v West Norfolk & Wisbech Area Health Authority [1986] AC 112 House of Lords.

Hart, B. and Risley, T. (1995) *Meaningful Differences in the Everyday Experience of Young American Children*. Baltimore, MD: Paul H. Brookes Publishing.

Jack, B.A., O'Brien, M.R., Kirton, J.A., Whelan, A., Baldry, C.R. and Groves, K.E. (2013) 'Enhancing communication with distressed patients, families and colleagues: the value of the Simple Skills Secrets model of communication for the nursing and healthcare workforce', *Nurse Education Today*, 33(2): 1550–6.

Johnson, M.H. (2005) 'Sensitive periods in functional brain development: problems and prospects', *Developmental Psychobiology*, 46(3): 287–92.

Kuo, D., Howtrow, A., Arango, P., Kaulthau, K., Simmons, J. and Neff, J. (2012) 'Family centred care: current applications and future directions in pediatric care', *Maternal and Child Health*, 16: 297–305.

Lambert, V. (2012) 'Theoretical foundations for communication', in V. Lambert, T. Long and D. Kelleher (eds), *Communication Skills for Children's Nurses*. Maidenhead: McGraw-Hill.

Lambert, V., Glacken, M. and McCarron, M. (2011) 'Communication between children and health professionals in a child hospital setting: a child transitional communication model', *Journal of Advanced Nursing*, 67(3): 569–82.

Mappa, P., Baverstock, A., Finlay, F. and Verling, W. (2010) 'Current practice with regard to "seeing adolescents on their own" during outpatient consultations', *International Journal of Adolescent Medicine and Health*, 22(2): 301–5.

McAndrew, S., Warne, T., Fallon, D. and Moran, P. (2012) 'Young, gifted and caring: a project narrative of young carers, their mental health and getting them involved in education, research and practice', *International Journal of Mental Health Nursing*, 21(1): 12–19.

Nursing and Midwifery Council (NMC) (2015) *The Code: Professional Standards of Practice and Behaviour for Nurses and Midwives*. London: NMC.

Roberts, J., Fenton, G. and Barnard, M. (2015) 'Developing effective therapeutic relationships with children, young people and their families', *Nursing Children and Young People*, 27(4): 30–5.

Robinson, S. (2010) 'Children and young people's views of health professionals in England', *Journal of Child Health*, 14(4): 310–26.

United Nations (1989) *Convention on the Rights of the Child* (UNCRC). London: UNICEF UK.

Van Staa, A.L. (2011) 'Unravelling triadic communication in hospital consultations with adolescents with chronic conditions: the added value of mixed methods research', *Patient Education and Counselling*, 82(3): 455–64.

Useful websites

Patient Opinion home page – www.patientopinion.org.uk/
The Children's Society home page – www.childrenssociety.org.uk

 To access further resources related to this chapter, visit the Values Exchange website at http://sagecomms.vxcommunity.com

9

Communicating with Middle-aged and Older People

Armin Luthi

• • • • • • • • • • • • Learning Objectives • • • • • • • • • • • •

By the end of this chapter, you will have developed an understanding of:

- features associated with ageing and contemporary society
- specific challenges in middle and older age
- overcoming stereotyping and stigma.

Don't forget to visit the Values Exchange website at http://sagecomms.vxcommunity.com for extra practice and revision activities.

• •

Introduction

> A human being would certainly not grow to be seventy or eighty years old if this longevity had no meaning for the species. The afternoon of human life must also have a significance of its own and cannot be merely a pitiful appendage to life's morning. (Carl Jung, cited in Moody, 2015, p. 29)

In this chapter, we will look at communication challenges with the mid- and older adult populations. Bear in mind that these are very generalised categorisations of age and, as shall be discussed, 'age' is not necessarily a stable concept. Ageing and the concepts of middle and older age will be defined and discussed. The nature of stigma and older people will form an important component of this chapter as often it is the stigmatising behaviour of society (including health professionals within that society) that becomes the most challenging issue for communicating with middle-aged and older adults. In fact, we do not recommend specific techniques for communicating with middle-aged and older adults as communication with these groups is no different from communication with other age groups. Instead, the emotional challenges affecting health associated with these periods of the lifespan will be discussed. Using practical critical thinking and mindfulness exercises, the chapter will encourage students to think about how to overcome stigmatising images and adapt their communication in the light of knowledge about these potential challenges.

Dementia is not discussed specifically in this chapter as we do not consider this to be the 'normal' consequence of age. Instead, communication with people with dementia is covered in the chapter on people with specific cognitive and communicative difficulties (Chapter 7).

Features associated with ageing in contemporary society

Middle adulthood is generally defined as approximately the 40s to the 60s. However, as noted above, concepts of age are fluid as perceptions are challenged and humans live longer with better environmental conditions. Some definitions specify 34–65 and indeed one of the authors remembers shuddering with horror when a student described them as middle-aged at the age of 34. However, 40–50 is normally considered the pathway to middle age (Wahl and Kruse, 2005).

Defining old age gets even more difficult. People are maintaining physical fitness for longer, aided by better living conditions. Yet, as we live longer, conditions associated with ageing such as cancer and dementia accompany longer lifespans. McCluskey (2013) suggests that some societies define age by characteristics rather than numbers. People are considered old when unable to inhabit the social roles previously held. Different age groupings see age differently. McCluskey (2013) points out that young students consider 50 to be old, yet people of that age in developed societies often do not consider themselves to be aged. The *Encyclopaedia Britannica* defines old age as 'the last stage of the normal lifespan' and notes that, whilst a changeable concept, it is generally assumed to commence around the age of 65 (www.britannica.com.science/old-age). However, 'normal' is variable, depending on biology, social structure and demography.

We live in an ageing world, but advances in medical and technical processes that reduce life-threatening illnesses and create better living conditions and environments mean that the mean age of the average citizen in the first world is now getting older all the time. In 1870, there were 1 million people over 65 in the USA and there are now 41.1 million. Life expectancy in the USA was 47 in 1900, and is now 79; 4% of the population were aged over 65 in 1900, and now it is 13.3% (Moody, 2015). Currently, there are 11.4 million people over 65 in the UK and 23.2 million over 50, so the numbers are set to rise (Age UK, 2015).

Whilst, on the one hand, this is good news, there have also been problems with how we look after our ageing population, with well-publicised concerns about neglect in care and nursing homes, and 'elder abuse' per se (Higgs and Gilleard, 2015; Moody, 2015). In line with more positive physical changes to the health status of an ageing population, there have been other, socio-cultural and psychological shifts that are more questionable. Exploration of the way western society looks at the process and 'acceptability' of ageing is necessary, and whether these attitudes, beliefs and stereotypes may be detrimental to middle-aged and older people, especially in terms of therapeutic care.

Ageing: an illness or a reality?

Over the last 50 or so years, there have been marked alterations in the way people are expected to present themselves, with youthful perfection increasingly seen as a 'norm' to which we should all aspire (Stuart-Hamilton, 2012). The trend for fad diets, cosmetic surgery and a rise in personal dissatisfaction mirror this (Moody, 2015). However, this emphasis on youthfulness and physical attractiveness rests very uneasily with the biological realities of ageing, and this has led to some psychological tension in a society that appears to have become less able to accommodate and accept the truth of ageing. Some theorists argue that this has then been reflected in the way that we care for our older people, and not always to the good (Brogden, 2001).

As nurses, it is guaranteed that you will be caring for older people. We live in a society that is ageing and has developed the medical technology to greatly increase the average lifespan of its members. However, this has not necessarily been reflected in a comparable quality of care, as older clients are extremely vulnerable to abuse and/or neglect from professional carers and nurses (Age UK, 2015). In addition, the many scandals about elder care have sadly demonstrated how vulnerable our older people can be. There are also wider, more pernicious, prevailing socio-cultural stereotypes. We live in a society that can be described as 'individualised', that emphasises personal entitlement, immediate gratification and perfection, with material, rather than spiritual, goals and values at its heart. We now have the medical technology to enable us to live longer, but it seems we expect our older people to remain 'young' as well, and we seem to regard ageing as wrong or pathological in some way, mainly because our materialist outlook cannot accommodate concepts of death or dying, so instead we avoid or deny them (Moody, 2015). Consequently, there is a tendency to avoid or deny the reality of ageing in much the same way. As nurses, you will need to reflect on these processes to ensure that you do not allow them to compromise your professional practice.

Student story 9.1: Difficulty in relating to older people

I really worry about looking so young. I'm expected to be knowledgeable and be able to give advice but I look young and I don't think patients older than me will take me seriously.

Visit the Values Exchange website at http://sagecomms.vxcommunity.com for a broader discussion on this Student story.

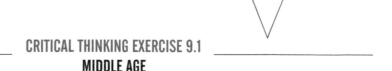

CRITICAL THINKING EXERCISE 9.1
MIDDLE AGE

Student nurses and midwives are often at the younger stage of adulthood. Spend five minutes writing down your understanding of what it means to be a person in middle age. What are the issues and themes that are significant to this group? What must it feel like to be a middle-aged person? Base your observations on your knowledge and experiences.

Specific challenges in middle and older age
Issues in mid-adulthood

This period may contain multiple psychological and social challenges. It is often described as the 'sandwich generation'. Allemand et al. (2015) discuss how multiple and complex challenges arise at this time of life. In middle age, people may be supporting both children and aged parents; they may be facing work-related problems such as changing jobs, real-ising that careers are stalling and experiencing life events such as location moves or relationship breakdown. It is also at this time that many middle-aged people feel they are giving out more practical, psychological and social support than they are receiving (Allemand et al., 2015). This can lead to social conflict and indeed to a retreat from social networks that could or should be offering support.

Lee-Baggley et al. (2005) note that personality traits may become more pronounced as ageing progresses. People who are introverted or extraverted will tend to respond to life events with exaggerated features of their already acquired personality traits. This can be adaptive or maladaptive; in particular, those who are introverted may be at risk of starting to become socially isolated in the wake of difficult life events. Allemand et al. (2015) found that those with a tendency towards neuroticism were least likely to report positive levels of social support in middle age.

This has implications for health as modern society's demands mean that we may live less socially connected lives than in previous times. Loneliness has become a topic of con-cern in current society:

> In the past, loneliness has been approached mainly from a cultural or social point of view, but work over the past decade by social neuroscientists such as John Cacioppo at the University of Chicago has provided scientific evidence of something many have long suspected: loneli-ness causes physiological events that wreak havoc on our health. (The Mental Health Foundation, 2010, p. 3)

Social isolation has an effect on stress hormones, is associated with health-damaging behaviour and has a generally deleterious impact on individual resilience. As discussed in Chapter 5, health behaviour has an important effect on health outcomes. Karran et al. (2011) found middle age to be the crucial point to develop obesity that could be problem-atic over time. Clearly, this is a period in which the practitioner could put the techniques of motivational interviewing and health behaviour change practice into effect (see Chapters 4 and 5).

The Mental Health Foundation (2010) also identifies middle age as the period of the lifespan with most potential for the development of social isolation. Yang and Victor (2008) note the importance of addressing creeping social isolation in middle age to pre-vent a worsening situation as people progress into older age. They advocate that societies should build structures that avoid contributing to the increase in potential for loneliness. The Mental Health Foundation (2010) urges health and social services to include an assessment of social isolation as part of general healthcare and to also consider measures to improve social connectedness as part of treatment, where relevant.

_____ CRITICAL THINKING EXERCISE 9.2 _____
NURSING MIDDLE-AGED PEOPLE

Using your thoughts, reflections and observations from the last mindfulness exercise, now spend five minutes writing down your understanding of the process of nursing middle-aged people. What are the clinical nursing issues and themes? What might be the challenges?

Issues for the older adult

_____ CRITICAL THINKING EXERCISE 9.3 _____
BEING AN OLDER ADULT

Student nurses and midwives are often at the younger stage of adulthood. Spend five minutes writing down your understanding of what it means to be a person in old age. What are the issues and themes that are significant to this group? What must it feel like to be an older person? Base your observations on your knowledge and experiences.

There are assumptions made about cognitive ability as ageing takes place. It was thought that intelligence peaked in adolescence and thereafter steadily declined (Santrock, 2013). Current research, however, points to an increasing vocabulary until much older age and to the development of differing types of intelligence as ageing progresses. Fluid intelligence – the ability to think creatively, to respond swiftly, etc. – is thought to build until the ages of 30 or 40, whilst crystallised intelligence builds up and increases over the following stages of the lifespan. Crystallised intelligence refers to stored lifetime experience and education, resulting in an increased vocabulary, the ability to use chemical/mathematical formulae and to use that stored experience to apply to problems. In addition, IQ scores are improving generation on generation due to improved nutrition and environmental circumstances. Moran (2012) discusses how older people can compensate for the decline in fluid intelligence if they have a good level of crystallised intelligence. Theory of mind – the ability to employ social understanding and to interact empathetically with others – has been tested across generations, and although there is consensus that the physical ageing process does result in declines in cognitive and social functioning, better health and education compensate for deficits (Duval et al., 2011). Self-esteem is also a factor. Robbins and Widaman (2012) found that those with good self-esteem in adolescence increased in self-esteem until the age of 50 and also had better health and life outcomes generally.

There are some specific communication problems that older people experience in healthcare situations. Many older adults have been found to ask fewer questions and consequently, too often, lack the information they require about their condition (Thompson et al., 2010). As they note, all healthcare practitioners should be competent to communicate across all age groups. Therefore, it may be necessary to make extra effort to check for understanding or to see if there are any unanswered questions. It might also be helpful to ensure a friend or family member accompanies the older person, if appropriate and acceptable to that older person. Whilst 'old' means something different today when compared to 20 years ago, it is still the case that a number of those in their 70s and beyond will start to find themselves requiring healthcare, and potentially for multiple co-existing conditions. Thompson et al. (2010) point out that in addition to their usual communicative competence, practitioners also need to consider the content of their communicative encounters with older adults. This includes diverse areas such as clinical awareness and questioning around potential multiple drug interactions, and social awareness around a non-patronising and collaborative approach.

Overcoming stereotyping and stigma

Stereotyping and stigma are possibly the most important barriers to effective communication with older people. There is no doubt that older people are heavily stereotyped in western society (Higgs and Gilleard, 2015; Moody, 2015). Stereotyping is a mental process by which we make very generalised and generic assumptions (often detrimentally) about people as *groups*, rather than as individuals (Stuart-Hamilton, 2012). In doing so, we take away the unique diversity and idiosyncrasies of any one individual person to replace them with a set of limited, highly predictable and generalised qualities that we ascribe to every member of the group who is being stereotyped (e.g. 'all adolescents are potential trouble makers').

These are cognitive *biases*, as we have discussed in previous chapters in Part 1 of this book, and, like all cognitive biases, they are designed to help us in how we manage sensory information via our perceptive processes. In other words, they help us to quickly and readily draw conclusions from situations in which there are many variables from which to choose (or, in other words, when there's a lot going on).

It is essential to remember that it can also very easily become destructive if we are not careful. It is vital to remember that once we are experiencing stress, our cognitive biases become increasingly narrow, inflexible and rigid. And so it is important to always be aware that, first, stereotyping is irrational, and, second, stereotyping swiftly leads to prejudice, and prejudice leads to conflict, dislike and hostility. Therefore, we must always remain aware of how easily we can all start stereotyping, especially when we are feeling stressed. Once we allow ourselves to unthinkingly stereotype, we start to discriminate and this leads to alienation and dehumanisation, and this can have catastrophic results, especially in care and nursing environments. For instance, a study by Liu et al. (2012) found that nurses held negative attitudes and believed in unhelpful stereotypes about ageing and the elderly that were anti-therapeutic. We have to acknowledge the impact that this has on nursing care for the elderly, as when these stereotypes go unchallenged, it can lead to abuse and neglect of the elderly, as happened at Stafford Hospital.

In Staffordshire in 2010, it was found that up to 1,200 more people died during 2005–08 than should have been expected whilst in the care of Stafford Hospital. In his report, Robert Francis QC noted that 'It was striking how many patients' accounts related to basic nursing care as opposed to clinical errors leading to injury or death' (Goodman, 2015). In essence, these patients were neglected to death, and they were all elderly.

CRITICAL THINKING EXERCISE 9.4
MID STAFFS PUBLIC INQUIRY

As a student nurse, it is essential that you read and understand the Francis Report. In this mindfulness exercise, review the key findings of the Francis Report (at http://webarchive.nationalarchives.gov.uk/20150407084003/http://www.midstaffspublicinquiry.com/report) and then reflect on the following questions:

- Do you think that this scandalous situation would have been allowed to continue for so long if the patients had been young adults or children?
- How might the situation have been different?
- And do you think nursing staff might have been less neglectful if they had been caring for a different type of client?

- What type of stereotyping led to this situation?
- And what especially do you think were the predominant stereotypes held about the elderly?

Visit the Values Exchange website at http://sagecomms.vxcommunity.com to develop your critical thinking skills and debate your thoughts and decisions.

As has already been noted, stereotypes predominate throughout our society. However, we, as qualified and educated healthcare professionals, have a duty of care to challenge and rectify these stereotypes to ensure that they do not negatively influence our attitudes, conduct or practice. Unfortunately, older people are especially at risk of unhelpful and negative stereotyping by public and professionals alike, so it is essential that we, as nurses, remain mindful that we are one of the groups who are prone to doing this. As Moody (2015) says, the concept, nature and process of ageing cause us to explore the very fundamentals of life, death and the meaning of our existence. And prior to the 20th century (with people dying on average at age 40–50), this question never really occurred in any real literal sense, as there were no elderly people. Now, of course, this is very different, and we, as a culture (and as a profession), are left struggling to make sense of this very complex (but very human) aspect of life. And, sadly, it has had some negative consequences, not least in our tendency to lack consistency in our care of and respect for older people.

Moody (2015) identifies a number of negative stereotypes common to the elderly; let's look at some of these, focusing on their validity, particularly as you are likely to hear them said in practice by nurses and other healthcare professionals.

CRITICAL THINKING EXERCISE 9.5
STEREOTYPE 1 – 'OLDER PEOPLE ARE ALL THE SAME'

There is a long-standing stereotype that older people lack individuality and are somehow a 'herd' to all be treated exactly the same rather than as unique individuals, each entitled to respect, compassion and consideration. Stuart-Hamilton (2012) highlights our readiness to believe this stereotype, and it is a deeply worrying one, given that this type of thinking gives us carte blanche to objectify and dehumanise the elderly without reflection.

Writers like Moody (2015) align this thinking to other wider social attitudes that see the elderly as a 'burden' who parasitically (and expensively) drain economic and physical resources at an alarming rate, and whose numbers are growing out of control.

What are your thoughts on this stereotype?

CRITICAL THINKING EXERCISE 9.6
STEREOTYPE 2 – 'OLDER PEOPLE ARE NATURALLY MORE CONSERVATIVE AND JUDGEMENTAL, MAKING IT HARD TO WORK THERAPEUTICALLY WITH THEM'

There is a long-standing stereotype that older people are more conservative and judgemental, and this is often presented as a natural and inevitable part of the ageing process. However, there is no

(Continued)

(Continued)

evidence for this, and, in fact, as the original rebellious teenagers of the 1950s and 1960s reach their 60s and 70s, it is in fact they who are rebelling against our conservative judgements by refusing to conform to our stereotypes of how we expect 'old people' to behave (Stuart-Hamilton, 2012). However, because we hold stereotypes about age-appropriate behaviour (and so expect our older people to be conservative, prudish and disapproving), we do not like it when they refuse to conform, and often label 'rebellious' older people as 'demented' or 'disordered' (Moody, 2015).

What are your thoughts on this stereotype?

CRITICAL THINKING EXERCISE 9.7
STEREOTYPE 3 – 'OLDER PEOPLE EXPERIENCE A MARKED DECLINE IN MENTAL FUNCTIONING AND ARE ALMOST LIKE SMALL CHILDREN'

There is often an assumption made amongst care and nursing staff that the 'best way' to treat older people is to patronise them, talking to them and treating them as though they were small children, usually from a stereotypical assumption that they have a reduced mental capacity (Moody, 2015). Again, this is not true, and evidence shows that cognitive functioning does not necessarily decline in older people (Stuart-Hamilton, 2012). But (as is true for people of *all* ages), it is essential that everyone is able to keep their minds active, challenged and stimulated in order to avoid intellectual decline. However, as many care and nursing environments offer little stimulation (because clients are 'too child-like'), the elderly *become institutionalised* instead, and so develop the apathy and dependency that come with institutionalisation (Moody, 2015). This institutionalisation is then labelled as 'childishness' by nursing and care staff, and so the malignant alienation seen at Stafford Hospital is born.

This is an example of iatrogenic care, where the care offered actually *causes* illness and decline (as per Stafford Hospital), showing how important it is for staff to challenge this type of stereotyping, as otherwise a carte blanche approach develops, focused on keeping senior clients in boring, sterile and unstimulating environments that *actually lead* to their cognitive decline, thus creating problems.

What are your thoughts on this stereotype?

CRITICAL THINKING EXERCISE 9.8
STEREOTYPE 4 – 'ALL THE OLD HAVE GOT TO LOOK FORWARD TO IS DETERIORATION AND DEATH, AND THEY JUST USE UP VALUABLE RESOURCES'

Western society has developed a deep unease with the whole concept of death that has led us to either avoid or deny it. Contemporary society has also lost its relationship with more ritualised and spiritual processes, relying on science and technology to hide death away from everyday life (Moody, 2015). And as the reality of death has become impersonal, bureaucratised and sterile, so we, as a society, have become detached and frightened of death (Moody, 2015). Because older people are a living embodiment of the inevitability of death, we have tried to treat them in the same way. And this has had an impact on how we see ageing in a number of complex ways.

What are your thoughts on this stereotype?

Patient story 9.1

Luckily my mother left hospital and stayed in a brilliant rehab care facility – she was extremely traumatised after her stay at ****** but is slowly recovering. If this is the way we are going to treat our older people it is very distressing – most of the issues were around basic nursing care and basic doctor attendance. Communication with concerned relatives who can see things going badly wrong should surely be a priority.

First, we have come to see ageing as a 'problem', not a stage of life; thus, we forget what ageing really represents – a part of life we will all face. And rather than a biological process alone, ageing

is a social phenomenon, an outcome of social evaluations of the older person's worth. Ageing itself – an inevitable process – is not a problem. Nor is it equivalent to an illness. A crude demographic determinism which sees the elderly as a problem is misconceived. It confuses a biological process – growing old – with the social and political factors that determine the treatment of the elderly. (Brogden, 2001, p. 13)

Second, we have lost an understanding of what Yen Chun et al. (2016) refer to as *gero-transcendence*, whereby ageing is regarded as a *natural and progressive* process of maturation and wisdom (and a state of mind that can only be reached by the ageing process itself). As nurses, it is essential that we embrace the values of gerotranscendence, as it sees ageing in a naturalistic and positive light, with older people as possessors of a special body of knowledge/wisdom that is unique to them. This in itself is a natural and healthy preparation for death and, as such, a spiritual process.

Critical debate 9.1

As nurses do we discriminate against older people? Do we communicate with older people differently?

Conclusion

This chapter has considered the problems of defining older age in contemporary society. It has examined some of the psychosocial factors that influence the lives of middle- and older-aged adults. However, it concludes that stigmatising and stereotyping are the most powerful issues facing older people and the professionals interacting with them. Consequently, much of the content focuses on inviting the student nurse to engage with exercises to acknowledge and explore prejudicial attitudes towards older people. As noted throughout Part 2 of this book, often there are no special techniques or secrets to effectively communicating with specific groups. Instead, it is about confronting the societal and individual cognitive biases held by the professionals. As always, where professionals can be mindful of their own emotions and actions, they can more effectively empathise and communicate compassionately with their patients.

References

Age UK (2015) *Your Rights at Work: Overview*. Available at: www.ageuk.org.uk/work-and-learning/discrimination-and-rights/your-rights-at-work/overview/ (accessed 16 April 2016).

Allemand, M., Scaffhuser, K. and Martin, M. (2015) 'Long-term correlated change between personality traits and perceived social support in middle adulthood', *Social and Psychological Bulletin*, 41(3): 420–32.

Brogden, M. (2001) *Geronticide*. London: Jessica Kingsley.

Duval, C., Piolino, P., Bejanin, A., Eustache, F. and Desgranges, B. (2011) 'Age effects on different components of theory of mind', *Consciousness and Cognition*, 20(3): 627–42.

Goodman, B. (2015) 'Why do nurses behave as they do?', 20 February. Available at: www.benny goodman.co.uk/why-do-nurses-behave-as-they-do/ (accessed 10 May 2016).

Higgs, P. and Gilleard, C. (2015) *Rethinking Old Age: Theorising the Fourth Age*. London: Palgrave Macmillan.

Karran, E., Mercken, M. and De Strooper, B. (2011) 'The amyloid cascade hypothesis for Alzheimer's disease: an appraisal for the development of therapeutics', *Nat. Rev. Drug Discov.*, 10: 698–712.

Lee-Baggley, D., Preece, M. and DeLongis, A. (2005) 'Coping with interpersonal stress: role of big five traits', *Journal of Personality*, 73: 1141–80.

Liu, Y., Norman, I. and White, A. (2012) 'Nurses' attitudes towards older people: a systematic review', *Nursing Studies*, 50(9): 1271–82.

McCluskey, K. (2013) *Lifespan Development*. London: Elsevier.

Mental Health Foundation (2010) *The Lonely Society*. Available at: www.mentalhealth.org.uk/publications/the-lonely-society (accessed 12 November 2015).

Moody, S. (2015) *Ageing: Concepts and Controversies*. London: Sage.

Moran, M. (2012) 'Lifespan development: the effects of typical aging on theory of mind', *Behavioural Brain Research*, 237: 32–40.

Robbins, W. and Widaman, K. (2012) 'Life-span development of self-esteem and its effects on important life outcomes', *Journal of Personality and Social Psychology*, 102(6): 1271–88.

Santrock, J. (2013) *Lifespan Development*. New York: McGraw-Hill.

Stuart-Hamilton, I. (2012) *The Psychology of Ageing*. London: Jessica Kingsley.

Thompson, T., Parrott, R. and Nussbaum, D. (2010) *The Routledge Handbook of Communication*. London: Routledge.

Wahl, H.-W. and Kruse, A. (2005) 'Historical perspectives on the lifespan', in S. Willis and M. Martin (eds), *Middle Adulthood*. London: Sage. pp. 1–34.

Yang, K. and Victor C.R. (2008) 'The prevalence for and risk factors for loneliness among older people', *Ageing and Society*, 28(3): 305–27.

Yen Chun, L., Wang, C.J. and Wang, J. (2016) 'Effects of a gerotranscendence educational program on gerotranscendence recognition, attitude towards aging and behavioral intention towards the elderly in long-term care facilities: a quasi-experimental study', *Nurse Education Today*, 36: 324–9.

Useful websites

Bronfenbrenner Centre for Translational Research, Cornell University on the lifespan – www.bctr. cornell.edu/

Encyclopaedia Britannica on old age – www.britannica.com/science/old-age

Mental Health Foundation home page – www.mentalhealth.org.uk/

Mid Staffs public inquiry – http://webarchive.nationalarchives.gov.uk/20150407084003/http://www.midstaffspublicinquiry.com/

To access further resources related to this chapter, visit the Values Exchange website at http:// sagecomms.vxcommunity.com

10

Integrating Mindful Communication Skills for Complex Encounters

Jean Shapcott

• • • • • • • • • • • Learning Objectives • • • • • • • • • • • •

By the end of this chapter, you will have developed an understanding of:

* working with distress and anger
* breaking bad news
* communication with people with life-limiting and end-of-life conditions.

 Don't forget to visit the Values Exchange website at http://sagecomms.vxcommunity.com for extra practice and revision activities.

• •

Introduction

Even nurses with the best and most effective communication skills can be challenged by difficult situations and interactions. The way in which they respond to these will depend on many factors, some related to the nurse, some to the patients and some to the situation or interaction itself. For example, every nurse brings their own personality, history, experiences and culture to every encounter with a patient and members of their family. Similarly, patients and relatives come to the encounter with their own backgrounds, whilst many are also experiencing some disruption to their normal functioning that may require readjusting, coping with and healing.

Instances where communication may be considered difficult include specific clinical situations and the sharing of specific diagnoses (Sheldon et al., 2006), for example following the intra-uterine death of a much wanted baby, communicating with patients whose cancer has metastasised or discussing the withdrawal of treatment at the end of a patient's life. Other components of difficult encounters may be related to the emotions experienced by nurses during their interactions with patients and relatives alongside the coping mechanisms employed to manage these. The challenges posed by the extensive communicative requirements for nurses, which have been explored throughout this book, can also contribute to difficult encounters, for example the need to maintain effective communication between members of the inter-professional team and the triad of communication characteristic of nursing children.

The stress of illness can evoke many emotions in patients and relatives which are often shared with nurses. Facilitating emotional expression and disclosure, as well as identifying coping mechanisms that are effective for patients and family members, are necessary components of the role of the nurse, however the emotions experienced, and often expressed, can make communication difficult. Negative emotions in both nurses and patients contribute to challenging situations and encounters. A nurse's ability to communicate effectively with patients and family members can be greatly affected by the feelings of hopelessness a nurse may be experiencing during withdrawal of treatment at the end of life, whilst communication can be particularly challenging when patients or relatives direct their negative emotions, particularly anger, at nurses. This chapter will explore how effective communication can be maintained in these difficult and complex situations.

Working with distress and anger

It is important to recognise that the engagement of nurses in communication can be affected by the emotional insecurity associated with challenging interactions. Nurses use varying degrees of connectedness and disconnectedness in order to maintain emotional control during interactions (Sheldon et al., 2006). They have described using distancing tactics because of fear that they will not be able to handle their own negative emotions, such as anxiety and distress, during difficult interactions. However, nurses who disconnect during challenging interactions with patients might further inhibit future communication with them, since failure to allow open communication and patient disclosure is likely to increase patient anxiety. It is clear that nurses' self-awareness regarding their personal emotional responses and the potential impact of these on effective communication strategies is crucial when considering patient outcomes.

It is often more productive to regard the encounter itself as difficult rather than perceive the patients themselves as problematic (Breen and Greenberg, 2010). Whilst recognising that particular patient behaviours may make a nurse feel uncomfortable, challenges may also lie in the setting, purpose and timing of the encounter between the nurse and the patient or relative. The Simple Skills Secrets model (Jack et al., 2013) has been referred to throughout Part 2 of this book.

Simple Skills Secret

1. Patient gives cue
2. Healthcare professional asks open question
3. Listening and using silence
4. Encouraging
5. Summarising
6. Assisting the formation of the patient's own plan
7. Whilst resisting the urge to rush in with a solution

This model enables nurses to respond to distress or unanswerable questions posed by patients or relatives without becoming involved in an interaction they are unable to handle. The key messages of this model are that nurses need to know how to open, maintain and close difficult encounters; that unanswerable questions are, by their very nature, impossible to answer, so the nurse should not attempt to do so; and that the individual (patient or relative) is the only one who knows or will recognise what the issues are, where the answers lie and is able to make a plan to manage them.

Encounters with angry patients are an unavoidable reality in nursing practice. It is likely that readers of this chapter will have experienced at least one, if not many, such interactions. The first time a nurse encounters an angry patient or relative may be more than simply challenging – it is likely to engender difficult emotions within the nurse and may even be frightening. However, despite our natural reactions to anger, it is not only destructive and damaging to the therapeutic relationship between the nurse and patient or relative, but can also lead to distrust on both sides (Chang, 2010).

CRITICAL THINKING EXERCISE 10.1
DEALING WITH ANGER

Consider a situation during which you were in the presence of someone who was angry. What do you think triggered their anger? How did you, or others who were present, respond to the person and their anger? Were your, or other people's, interventions successful in reducing their anger?

 Visit the Values Exchange website at http://sagecomms.vxcommunity.com to develop further and debate your thoughts and decisions.

When considering interactions with angry or distressed people, it is important to remember the possible sources of their anger or distress as this may aid effective communication with them. Anger with aggression is often a sign of anxiety, grief or even feelings of guilt and is a common response either to a change in someone's health status, which may have serious implications for their future wellbeing, or to previous healthcare encounters which might have been perceived as unsatisfactory (Breen and Greenberg, 2010). According to Chang (2010), the natural history of anger entails five stages:

1. Predisposition
2. Irritation
3. Escalation
4. Outburst
5. Consequence(s)

Chang advocates a simple strategy for communicating with angry patients and relatives – the five As of anger deflection:

1. Allow
2. Absorb
3. Assess
4. Acknowledge
5. Absolve

Once the individual has indicated their anger through a verbal or non-verbal cue, it is important to *allow* the individual to vent their anger without interruption in a setting where privacy is assured and the likelihood of being disturbed is minimal. This necessitates the nurse having enough time to listen, and recognising that, whilst listening is important, so also is being seen to respond in an appropriate manner (Breen and Greenberg, 2010). The nurse should invite the individual to raise all their concerns and only interrupt if this is absolutely essential for clarification purposes. This is important, since, even if the nurse believes that a situation has been misunderstood or that the individual's responses are clearly incorrect or inappropriate, any interruption is likely to be perceived as defensive and carries the risk of aggravating an already difficult situation. Allowing the individual to vent in this manner can quickly limit the harsh tone of the encounter and may even prevent further escalation (Chang, 2010).

After the individual has expressed their concerns, the nurse should *absorb* the experience with a moment of silence. Any words from the nurse at this stage will sound either antagonistic or defensive to the angry person. This is one of the most important strategies during an angry encounter, but also the most simple. Silence provides the nurse with an opportunity to categorise the individual's concerns in their mind and gives the angry person time and space to think (Chang, 2010; Jack et al., 2013).

Chang (2010) indicates that the next step is to remind the individual of the purpose of the encounter in terms of their health and wellbeing and undertake a nursing *assessment*. He suggests that any potential breakdown in the therapeutic relationship between the individual and the nurse can be redressed by this simple focus on the individual and their needs, through which key problems can be anticipated and processed with the aim of generating an effective response.

The Simple Skills Secret model (Jack et al., 2013) recognises the importance of summarising the interaction in one or two salient points when *acknowledging* the individual's outburst. This enables the nurse to establish some common ground by accepting the individual's right to be angry, whilst pointing out the potential effect that the outburst might have on future care and interactions with healthcare staff (Chang, 2010). At this point, screening questions (Jack et al., 2013) facilitate a further exploration of issues to ensure that the individual feels all their concerns have been voiced. It is very tempting, once all the individual's concerns have been expressed, for the nurse to step in with things they believe might help, but it is important, as part of acknowledgement, to emphasise the individual's active role in ensuring the encounter is both satisfying and constructive. It is therefore helpful to encourage the individual to consider their own solutions to the concerns they have raised, thereby avoiding long, in-depth conversations for which the nurse may feel unprepared, unskilled or short of time.

In this way, *absolution* (Chang, 2010) can be achieved. Excellent nursing care will have been provided despite the challenging nature of the situation. The nurse will not have taken on the issues raised by the individual, which are not theirs to address, and will not feel responsible for solutions which only the individual themself can address (Jack et al., 2010). Instead, common ground will have been established between the nurse and the individual who has been empowered to address their own concerns (Chang, 2010).

<hr>

CRITICAL THINKING EXERCISE 10.2
ANGER

How do you feel now about encountering an angry patient or relative? Do you see how this strategy might enable you to interact with them in a more productive and satisfying manner? Are there any aspects of the five As of anger deflection or the Simple Skills Secrets model that are particularly salient for you? Are there any elements which you are now aware that you need to work on? For example, how comfortable are you with silence in patient interactions?

<hr>

Breaking bad news

Breaking bad news is another example of a potentially difficult encounter with patients and families. Bad news can be considered as any news that drastically and negatively alters an individual's view of their future (Buckman, 1985). An individual's experience of such news is dependent on their concept of time and future as well as their capacity for abstract thinking, which, for some patients and family members (e.g. children), may be limited. It is therefore essential that any new information given to an individual makes sense to them and fits in with their current understanding and experience of life (Tuffrey-Wijne and Watchman, 2015).

The most commonly held view is that all patients should be told the truth about their condition, clearly demonstrating application of the ethical principle of autonomy (Munoz-Sastre et al., 2012). Most patients want to be told about their illness, treatment and prognosis whether the news is good or bad (Warnock et al., 2010). A less common, protectionist view is that patients should not be told anything unless they themselves express concern, in which case the principle of non-maleficence would be applied and part of the truth would be told (Munoz-Sastre et al., 2012). This is often seen in situations where the patient is a child, has a learning disability or some other condition resulting in a limited capacity to understand information. However, time will not change what has to be said or done, therefore there is no benefit to the patient or their relatives in postponing or finding reasons to delay giving bad news (Crawford et al., 2013), and doing so might actually lead to distrust and a feeling of being deceived.

Breaking bad news is a process involving interactions which occur before, during and after the moment at which the information is shared. There is growing evidence that assimilation of bad news is slow and incremental (Griffiths et al., 2015), and therefore this process is a complex and highly skilled activity that needs to be done well to minimise detrimental effects on the patient, their relatives and future relationships with healthcare professionals. Whilst it is predominantly doctors who break bad news, the process is also a multi-disciplinary activity which requires the active involvement of a range of professionals working together as a team. It is important to recognise that long-lasting distress, confusion and resentment may occur when bad news is not imparted well (Warnock et al., 2010).

CRITICAL THINKING EXERCISE 10.3
REFLECT ON RECEIVING BAD NEWS

Spend five minutes reflecting on an occasion when you received bad news. If you believe you have never been in such a situation, consider something you may have seen on TV/video or have witnessed in placement:

- What was the nature of the bad news?
- Who broke the bad news?
- Where did this take place?
- How did you or the individual receiving the news react?
- How did the person breaking the bad news manage this reaction?

A number of barriers to the effective delivery of bad news have long been acknowledged. Healthcare professionals may be concerned about upsetting people, but it has already been noted that most patients want to know about their condition and these concerns may, in reality, reflect the lack of training that many healthcare professionals receive in breaking bad news and their consequent fears regarding being able to cope with their own and patients'/relatives' emotional responses. Other barriers include the lack of time and privacy for such encounters as well as potential language and/or cultural barriers between the healthcare professional and the patient. In some situations, it is also important to recognise that there may be a discrepancy between the wishes of the patient and those of their relatives as to whether information should be shared or withheld, and to consider the reasons behind these (Warnock et al., 2010).

Patient story 10.1: Carly

Carly is a 15-year-old girl who was diagnosed three years ago with Acute Lymphoblastic Leukaemia. She longs to be able to do normal 'teenage' things, but is exhausted by treatment and fed up with being in pain. After three cycles of chemotherapy, doctors have told her father Daniel, who is a lone parent, that the treatment has not been successful and that Carly is going to die. Daniel is adamant that he does not want his daughter to know her prognosis. However, Carly is aware that the doctors have talked to Daniel and that he seems very sad. She has also sensed a change in the way in which her nurses on the ward approach her and she asks you directly 'Am I dying?':

1   Why might Daniel have taken this decision?
2   In light of Carly's age and by applying communication, nursing and ethico-legal principles, how would you respond to Carly's question?

Nurses undertake a number of supportive activities when patients and their relatives receive bad news. These include clarifying and explaining what has been said to patients and relatives by doctors, assessing their needs for additional information and helping them to cope with their emotional reactions (Warnock et al., 2010). Since nurses' engagement in the process can occur at any point in a patient's journey, this engagement tends to occur on an ad hoc basis and at opportunistic moments. This may present many challenges to nurses, including being presented with unexpected questions without time to prepare an answer, an expectation that they will continue to work in close contact with the patient and relatives without time to de-brief or reflect, and time constraints due to workload demands.

A number of models have been developed to support and guide nurses engaged in breaking bad news (see Tables 10.1, 10.2 and 10.3).

Models of breaking bad news

All the models indicate the need to plan ahead whenever possible. This necessitates preparing the environment to ensure privacy and prevent interruption, and preparing yourself and the recipient(s) of the news. Preparing the patient and their relatives for information that needs to be shared and ensuring that they fully understand that they need to hear this news is a key component of the process. It is important that jargon, elaborate reasons or

Table 10.1   ABCDE model

Advance preparation – time/privacy	Confirm medical facts
	Prepare emotionally for the encounter
Building a therapeutic relationship	Identify patient preferences
Communicating well	Determine existing knowledge/understanding
	Proceed at patient's/relatives' pace
	Avoid medical jargon and euphemisms
	Allow for silence and tears
	Answer questions
Dealing with patient and family reactions	Assess and respond
	Empathise
Encouraging/validating emotions	Offer realistic hope
	Deal with own emotional need

Source: Rabow and McPhee (1999)

Table 10.2   SPIKES protocol

Setting	Setting up the interview; involves planning and preparation
Perception	Assessing patient's/relatives' understanding
Invitation	Obtaining patient's/relatives' invitation to offer information
Knowledge	Delivering knowledge and information in a sensitive and timely way
Emotions	Addressing the emotions of the patient/relative using a person-centred approach
Strategy	Summarising and planning a future strategy

Source: Hagerty et al. (2005)

Table 10.3   RCN model

Preparation	Of self, recipient and environment
Communication	Delivery of the information
Planning	Agreeing what happens next
Follow-up	Documentation
	Provision of written information
	Liaison with other agencies

Source: Royal College of Nursing (2013)

euphemisms are avoided and that the temptation to rush over particularly upsetting or distressing elements of the news is resisted. Information should be given in small 'chunks' to avoid overloading the patient or relative and their understanding should be ensured before moving on to the next part of the information.

Ideally, those breaking bad news should take their lead regarding the pace of information delivery from the patient and their relatives. However, some individuals may absorb the information quickly and attempt to move the encounter forward at their pace, leaving others behind in their understanding. Sensitivity is essential to ensure the communication needs of all those involved are met with the provision of frequent summaries and the appropriate use of eye contact in order to engage all parties and ensure balanced information is given and an equal basis of understanding is achieved (Crawford et al., 2013).

Additional components of the nurse's communication toolkit when involved in breaking bad news include silence, permitting expression and touch. The importance of silence has been noted earlier in this chapter and a pause in the interaction can give patients and relatives time to absorb and assimilate information, so nurses should resist the temptation to rush in to fill the perceived void with more words. Silence does not imply a failure in communication; it suggests that information is being processed.

People react to bad news in a variety of ways, including some that nurses might perceive to be inappropriate, for example shame, humour and even laughter (Crawford et al., 2013). Although a nurse may find witnessing such cathartic moments challenging, they are a key component of the process. Patients and relatives may need explicit permission to express these emotions. A nurse can give this by acknowledging that the news was difficult to hear and hard to take in, whilst reassuring them that some people will feel angry, cry or express some other strong feelings.

Touch and proximity must be used with caution, but can provide extremely effective communication skills when breaking bad news. Some patients and relatives welcome physical contact, whilst others shy away from such intimacy with strangers. Touch is an invasion of interpersonal space and is open to cultural interpretation, so it is important that the nurse does not assume that their own conventions regarding these elements of communication are shared by the patient/relative receiving the bad news.

Breaking bad news is never easy, but it is an important aspect of communication in any field of nursing. What constitutes bad news for a child (for example, the loss of a favourite toy) may seem trivial in comparison to a young adult who has been told they have a life-limiting illness, but it is important to refer back to the definition of bad news and recognise that the way in which the information given is perceived is entirely dependent on the individual receiving it, since only they know the impact it will have on their future life. A nurse must also remember that the delivery of bad news is not the end of that patient's healthcare journey and that ongoing communication is essential.

Communicating with people with life-limiting and end-of-life conditions

Guidelines related to caring for people whose condition is life limiting or who are approaching the end of their lives identify sensitive communication between healthcare professionals, the patient and those they consider important to them as a key priority (National Institute for Health and Care Excellence, 2015), in order that their involvement in decision making and advanced care planning might be successfully facilitated. Communication is often viewed as the primary intervention as patients approach the end of their lives (Norton et al., 2013). Limited communication can lead to poor decision making and patient outcomes with patients and relatives receiving sub-optimal care (Barnes et al., 2012).

It is recognised that so-called 'prognostic uncertainty' adds to the challenges of communicating with patients and relatives in this situation, since it is generally impossible patient is still in the pre-contemplation phase, may be unhelpful, and more successful when they have moved onto preparation. If relapse is seen as a natural occurrence rather than as a catastrophe, it becomes easier to move back into contemplation and begin the cycle again.

Motivational interviewing techniques allow the professional to engage with the natural ambivalence and resistance experienced by patients who would benefit from behaviour change. The practitioner explores ambivalence, the pros and cons of taking a course of action, avoids confrontation where there is resistance (this is a natural part of the process), and supports and helps build confidence once the patient has made the change (Mason, 2005).

CRITICAL THINKING EXERCISE 5.4
MOTIVATIONAL INTERVIEWING

Think of a situation where someone would benefit from changing their health behaviour and consider how you could engage them by using motivational interviewing techniques.

Pre-contemplation: How could you raise awareness about the risks involved in current unhealthy behaviour? Remember, your place is not to be critical or blame but to provide information about harm reduction.

Comtemplation: How could you help the patient to explore their ambivalence? What are the advantages and disadvantages of changing current behaviour? How might life get better? Would things feel worse in the short term? What could happen over the longer term? For example: What would be different in your life if you lost weight? Ask open-ended questions to encourage the patient to talk.

Preparation and Action: How can you work with the patient to set realistic and achievable goals? Check if you both understand each other. Are their differences between the goals and the current situation? If so, point these out. Make it clear that you are trying to understand the situation from their perspective, for instance 'Let me check that what you are saying is ... have I got that right?'

Maintenance: What tactics can both of you devise to help the patient stick to the planned behaviour change? Use positive statements to show you understand how well they are doing, despite the reality that behaviour change is difficult. Reflect back with the patient, using their words to look at progress as this can help them understand their motivation.

Relapse: *Relapse is normal.* Both you and the patient can accept this. It is not a disaster. Work with the patient to understand this and that you simply restart the process.

It is possible to incorporate motivational interviewing techniques into normal interaction with service users and patients. This may take a little more time, but as NICE (2015) and the UK House of Commons Health Committee (2014) note, it is imperative for health services to provide more effective communication with patients with long-term conditions to achieve better outcomes.

to predict the course of an illness or the exact timing of death (Broom et al., 2014). Effective communication is critically important (Walzack et al., 2013). Some healthcare professionals favour a 'softly softly' approach to discussions in these situations. Whilst this may have a short-term interpersonal gain since patients and relatives are likely to be less distressed, it also has long-term limitations since it may result in limited acceptance and acknowledgement of the reality of the situation (Broom et al., 2014).

Nurses should maintain a calm and open manner in all interactions with these patients and their relatives. Person-centred communication in which the latter are treated as individuals, and nurses are sensitive to their specific needs, is crucial since patients perceive a caring healthcare professional to be one who is both able and willing to meet the needs of individuals (Janssen and McLeod, 2010). Patients and relatives feel more at ease when nurses give them careful attention, seek common ground and provide care according to their expressed preferences, which can only be identified when nurses modify their communication approaches to explore and adapt to these wishes (Norton et al., 2013).

Nurses who actively listen to and are comfortable simply 'being with' patients and relatives allow them to reflect and explore their thoughts and emotions about their situation (Hawthorn, 2015). This is another instance where silence is a powerful and dynamic method of demonstrating support. However, any interaction with someone who has a life-limiting illness or is receiving palliative/end-of-life care requires both the nurse and the patient to be ready to engage in discussions about prognosis, palliative care and the end of life. For the patient, this means that the desire to know facts overrides any fear or ambivalence about discussing these issues, whilst nurses need to be comfortable, confident and able to talk about death and dying (Walzack et al., 2013).

CRITICAL THINKING EXERCISE 10.4
DEATH AND DYING

Once again, take five minutes to consider:

- How comfortable are you in talking about death and dying?
  Can you identify any factors that might have influenced your level of comfort?
- Now consider how such discussion might vary according to the patient (e.g. child/adult/person with a learning disability or mental health issue), setting (e.g. hospital ward/patient's own home), etc.

In such encounters, control over the discussion should actively be given to the patient. However, the nurse should be prepared to take the lead in raising complex or difficult subjects, for example prognosis or end-of-life care, as necessary. It is crucial that the nurse is honest about the patient's situation, acknowledging and explaining uncertainty where it exists, and balancing honesty with the patient's need to maintain hope (Norton et al., 2013). Despite the reality that care options in life-limiting illness may be limited or that current care cannot meaningfully improve survival chances or even enhance a patient's quality of life, the ability to enhance a patient's or relative's ability to maintain hope is a key element in ensuring the psychological wellbeing of patients and the ongoing therapeutic relationship (Broom et al., 2014; Hawthorn, 2015).

In this context, hope is a wide and multi-dimensional phenomenon and can hold different meanings for different people (Clayton et al., 2005). It can be perceived as the confident yet uncertain expectation of a future good that appears realistically possible and is personally significant for an individual. This sense of hope can be maintained if, once the nature of the condition or prognosis has been effectively communicated, the patient and relatives are offered some positive aspects of their future, for example the opportunity to continue to study for important examinations or effective pain management. However, both false promises and being too blunt in delivering information can effectively obliterate hope. In addition, hope can be easily eroded by negative messages from healthcare professionals, whether delivered verbally or non-verbally.

Patient story 10.2: Aaron

Aaron is 32 years old. He started drinking alcohol in his late teens when his parents' relationship broke down, finding that alcohol obliterated the emotions he was experiencing. His drinking increased significantly over subsequent years and was responsible for his relationship with his long-term partner coming to an end three years ago. As a result, he has not seen his two children since the break-up.

After several bouts of severe abdominal pain, which doctors at the walk-in centre attributed to pancreatitis, Aaron has recently been diagnosed with stage 4 cancer of the head of the pancreas, which is inoperable. He remains on an acute medical ward, having been referred to the palliative care team who are seeking a place for him in the local hospice. Since his diagnosis, Aaron has noticed that some nurses, who used to chat a lot and with whom he often shared a joke, are ignoring him. Others have stopped using his name, referring to him only as 'Bed 6'. Yet others seem to be constantly busy with no time to communicate with him. This morning, he overheard a conversation on the ward round: 'There is no question – his cancer is due to his drinking. Purely self-inflicted. Patients like him make me so angry – someone who really needs care could have that bed and we would then not be wasting our resources.' The response had been: 'He'll be dead soon – a painful death and, hopefully, quick.'

All the positive words from the few nurses who still seem to care for him now seem as nothing:

- Identify the factors in this scenario that will limit Aaron's ability to maintain hope.
- How might the nurses seek to facilitate him to adopt a more positive approach to his illness trajectory?

We hope you will not encounter a situation such as that described above, but, as discussed throughout this book, fear, ignorance and a lack of mindfulness can lead to a judgemental or evasive approach. Knowledge and preparation for communicating with patients with end-of-life conditions are important and necessary components of healthcare education.

Ballesteros, Centeno and Arandzamendi (2014) carried out a study with student nurses to explore the impact of education around palliative care. Students expressed their views on how the course had helped to overcome their fears (see Student story 10.1).

Student story 10.1: Student voices

'To overcome the fear of death by talking naturally about it' (NUR-So 120).

'Because sooner or later it will be our turn, and we have to begin to deal with it and also teach people how to deal with death as a natural event' (NUR-So 19). (Ballesteros et al., 2014, p. 3)

'It helped me to deal with my personal problems because I realised that grief is something that it is necessary' (NUR-So 68).

'To better understand situations experienced in the past' (NUR-Na 29).

'I have learned to put myself in other people's shoes, more so than from a simply physical or pathological perspective' (NUR-So 127).

'To know how to behave with a terminally ill person and try to understand' (NUR-So123).

'It has helped me to understand that communication and listening are the most important elements' (NUR-So 2).

'To learn that not only is the art of curing people important, but so is taking care of them' (NUR-So 88). (Ballesteros et al., 2014, p. 4)

Critical debate 10.1

Does healthcare education spend enough time on how to deal with the difficult and non-curable situations? Are you prepared?

Conclusion

This chapter has explored some of the more complex and difficult areas of communication in nursing. Key points to take away from this are that when interacting with an angry patient, active listening and a calm, structured approach are the key to successful communication; defensive or confrontational approaches will simply inflame the situation further; breaking bad news can be seen as a process in which nurses are involved at various stages – a number of models exist to guide and support nurses when engaged in breaking bad news, but it is important to maintain a person-centred, individual approach to these encounters; and in order to communicate effectively with patients who have life-limiting illnesses or are receiving palliative or end-of-life care, nurses must explore their own feelings about discussing death and dying in order to be ready to engage in such interactions. In addition, the ability to foster hope in patients and relatives is very important.

References

Ballesteros, M., Centeno, C. and Arantzamendi, M. (2014) 'A qualitative exploratory study of nursing students' assessment of the contribution of palliative care learning', *Nurse Education Today*, 34(6): 1–6.

Barnes, S., Gott, M., Chady, B., Seamark, D. and Halpin, D. (2012) 'Enhancing patient–professional communication about end-of-life issues in life-limiting conditions: a critical review of the literature', *Journal of Pain and Symptom Management*, 44(6): 866–79.

Breen, K.J. and Greenberg, P.B. (2010) 'Difficult physician–patient encounters', *International Medicine Journal*, 40(10): 682–8.

Broom, A., Kirby, E., Goad, P., Woolton, J. and Adams, J. (2014) 'The troubles of telling: managing communication about the end of life', *Qualitative Health Research*, 24(2): 151–62.

Buckman, R. (1985) 'Breaking bad news – why is it still so difficult?', *British Medical Journal*, 6430: 1597–9.

Chang, P.T.C. (2010) 'How I manage encounters with angry patients', *Medical Economics*, 87(10): 33–6.

Clayton, J.M., Butow, P.M., Arnold, R.M. and Tattersall, M.H. (2005) 'Fostering coping and nurturing hope when discussing the future with terminally ill cancer patients and their caregivers', *Cancer*, 103(9): 1965–75.

Crawford, D., Corkin, D., Coad, J. and Hollis, R. (2013) 'Educating children's nurses for communicating bad news', *Nursing Children and Young People*, 25(8): 28–33.

Griffiths, J., Ewing, G., Wilson, C., Connolly, M. and Grande, G. (2015) 'Breaking bad news about transitions to dying: a qualitative exploration of the role of the district nurse', *Palliative Medicine*, 29(2): 138–46.

Hagerty, R.G., Butow, P.N. and Ellis, P.M. (2005) 'Communicating with realism and hope: incurable cancer patients' views on the disclosure of prognosis', *Journal of Clinical Oncology*, 23(6): 1278–88.

Hawthorn, M. (2015) 'The importance of communication in sustaining hope at the end of life', *British Journal of Nursing*, 24(13): 702–5.

Jack, B.A., O'Brien, M.R., Kirton, J.A., Marley, K., Whelan, A., Baldry, C.R. and Groves, K.E. (2013) 'Enhancing communication with distressed patients, families and colleagues: the value of the Simple Skills Secrets model of communication for the nursing and healthcare workforce', *Nurse Education Today*, 33(12): 1550–6.

Janssen, A.L. and McLeod, R.D. (2010) 'What can people approaching death teach us about how to care?', *Patient Education*, 81(2): 251–6.

Munoz-Sastre, M.T., Sorum, P.C. and Mullett, E. (2012) 'Lay people's and health professionals' views about breaking bad news to children', *Child: Care, Health and Development*, 40(1): 106–14.

National Institute for Health and Care Excellence (NICE) (2015) *Care of Dying Adults in the Last Days of Life*. Available at: www.nice.org.uk/guidance/ng31 (accessed 12 January 2016).

Norton, S.A., Metzger, M., DeLuca, J., Alexander, S.C., Quill, T.E. and Gramling, R. (2013) 'Palliative care communication: linking patients' prognoses, values and goals of care', *Research in Nursing and Health*, 36(6): 582–90.

Rabow, M.W. and McPhee, S.J. (1999) 'Beyond breaking bad news: how to help patients who suffer', *Western Journal of Medicine*, 171(4): 260–3.

Royal College of Nursing (RCN) (2013) *Breaking Bad News: Supporting Parents when they are Told of their Child's Diagnosis – RCN Guidance for Nurses, Midwives and Health Visitors*. London: RCN. Available at: www2.rcn.org.uk/__data/assets/pdf_file/0006/545289/004471.pdf (accessed 16 April 2016).

Sheldon, L.K., Barrett, R. and Ellington, L. (2006) 'Difficult communication in nursing', *Journal of Nursing Scholarship*, 38(2): 141–7.

Tuffrey-Wijne, I. and Watchman, K. (2015) 'Breaking bad news to people with learning disabilities and dementia', *Learning Disability Practice*, 18(7): 16–23.

Walzack, A., Butow, P.N., Davidson, P.M., Bellemore, F.A., Tattersall, M.H.N., Clayton, J.M., et al. (2013) 'Patient perspectives regarding communication about prognosis and end-of-life issues: how can it be optimised?', *Patient Education and Counseling*, 90(3): 307–14.

Warnock, C., Tod, A., Foster, J. and Soreny, C. (2010) 'Breaking bad news in inpatient clinical settings: role of the nurse', *Journal of Advanced Nursing*, 66(7): 1543–55.

Useful websites

Macmillan Cancer Support home page – www.macmillan.org.uk/
National Council for Palliative Care on palliative care – www.ncpc.org.uk/palliative-care-explained
Palliative Care Guidelines – http://book.pallcare.info/
Supportive & Palliative Care (British Medical Journals) – http://spcare.bmj.com

 To access further resources related to this chapter, visit the Values Exchange website at http://sagecomms.vxcommunity.com

CONCLUSION TO

PART 2

Part 2 explored communication with a variety of different care groups. It sought to emphasise that, in most cases, the same set of skills and techniques can be adapted to fit the context of the individual within that care group. The Simple Skills Secret can be adapted to any anxious or distressed service user. The principles of motivational interviewing can be applied to any situation where health promotion and behaviour change are required.

Chapter 5 focused on groups of patients/service users where it is acknowledged that health professional communication could be much improved: those where 'difficult conversations' need to be had and for those with long-term conditions, requiring behavioural change. We suggested that alongside an empathic attitude, relatively simple techniques can enable the professional to communicate effectively and compassionately.

Chapter 6 concentrated on the group of service users who might (and do) argue that they face the most stigma in society and also from services supposed to care for them. This chapter pointed out that the same communicative techniques are as appropriate here as for any other care group. The major challenge is overcoming stigmatising attitudes.

Chapter 7 explored communication issues with those who have been born with or acquired some form of brain injury, necessitating particular forms of communication to be used.

Chapter 8 examined the specific features around children, families and young people that affect communication. It provided the context around the developmental needs of children and young people and suggested methods for appropriate communication.

Chapter 9 looked at the issues for middle-aged and older adults, again, very much like Chapter 6, noting the specific features of stigma and stereotyping.

Chapter 10 concluded Part 2 with an examination of those parts of healthcare often avoided or not spoken about: where the end point is not cure but rather someone has a life-limiting condition

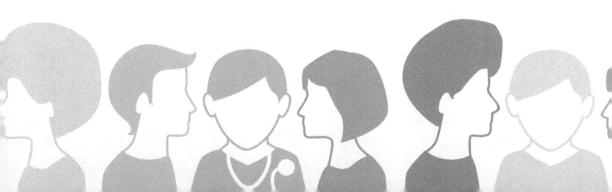

or one requiring palliative care. This chapter stressed the need for good levels of knowledge and preparation for this sensitive area of care, pointing out how communication can be carried out in a helpful and caring manner.

In conclusion, there are often psychosocial and other contextual factors that influence the patient or service user: fear, environmental setting, stage of life and, too often, being part of a stigmatised group. Therefore, to communicate effectively and compassionately, those factors need to be addressed. The student nurse or midwife can adapt their communication accordingly in the light of knowledge about the individual's need. Part 2 strongly suggested that all of us need to confront and challenge any stereotypical beliefs as it is these that often negatively influence our communicative interactions.

PART 3

EQUIPPING FOR THE FUTURE: THEORETICAL AND ETHICAL ISSUES

Part 3 of this book focuses on the transition to becoming a qualified professional. Consequently, the subject matter shifts from how to communicate compassionately to issues of thinking more deeply about the challenges facing newly qualified professionals. Chapter 11 looks at behaviour and thinking within organisations. Health services are generally delivered within organisational settings. Students tend to move on after a maximum 12-week (often shorter) placement. However, on taking up their first post, the newly qualified professional will have to negotiate the particular organisational culture, whilst, at the same time, demonstrating their fledgling leadership skills. Many ex-students (including one of the authors) find this period testing, so examination of the thinking and behaviours that help facilitate effective communicative functioning is necessary.

Chapter 12 examines one of the most worrying but common problems with work that involves 'emotional labour'. Burnout, more properly described as 'moral disengagement', is a risk factor for those in professions who are regularly confronted with difficult emotional situations. The transition period from student to professional is a significant period where student ideals may be shed as a (mistakenly) protective shield against the stresses of reality. Chapter 12 looks at the more constructive mechanisms for looking after oneself, in order to be able to look after others. Reflection and clinical supervision (in whatever form) are urged in order for practitioners to value themselves and to acknowledge the need for support in emotionally demanding areas.

Chapter 13 then goes on to conclude the book by suggesting that thinking about theory and reflection can enable us to move forward, both personally and professionally. Any number of relevant theorists/theories could be selected but we have chosen to focus on certain theories on ethical practice, collaborative communication and reflective theory.

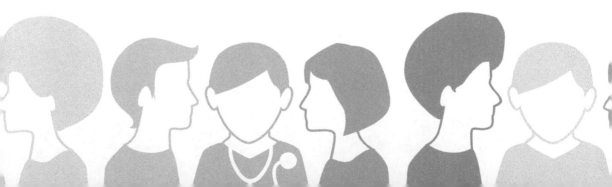

11

Communicating Authentically in Organisations

Judith Francois

• • • • • • • • • • • • • Learning Objectives • • • • • • • • • • • • •

By the end of this chapter, you will have developed an understanding of

- organisations, culture, communication and leadership
- the importance of self in leadership
- authentic self and authentic leadership.

Don't forget to visit the Values Exchange website at http://sagecomms.vxcommunity.com for extra practice and revision activities.

• •

Introduction

As students approach qualification, there is a need to consider communication from the perspective of working within an organisation and also in terms of their leadership role as a professional. As people progress within their chosen profession, there will be an imperative to develop one's own ability and to lead others in compassionate and communicative practice. This chapter provides the opportunity to consider the nature of communication in an organisation, and will also provide insight into the range of issues that can occur when this is lacking. The first sections will give a brief overview of organisational culture and leadership. The impact of organisational culture on patient care will be discussed, allowing individuals to appreciate how they might influence good practice. The latter sections are concerned with exploring the nature of 'authentic leadership' and unpicking the communicative behaviours required for leading in this manner.

Student story 11.1: Return to Gemma

Gemma is a student child field nurse in her third year, approaching qualification. She has really enjoyed her course and still loves interacting with the children. To some extent, she has gotten over her fears of 'looking too young' and thinks she can communicate pretty well with parents now. Her clinical skills are not bad, if she says so herself (her practice assessment documents do back this up). Feedback on her communication skills has also been very good and she feels confident in this type of communication.

However, whilst this is all positive, it isn't enough, she realises, as qualification looms. As Gemma prepares for interviews for her first job, she recognises that she is also going to have to be a leader/manager. She loves nursing but is not terribly comfortable at the thought of delegating and allocating tasks to others. She has observed other newly qualified staff struggling to cope with asking others to do things and wonders how she can better prepare herself. Can she lead others successfully?

 Visit the Values Exchange website at http://sagecomms.vxcommunity.com for a broader discussion on Gemma's story.

Patient story 11.1: Impact of poor communication and organisation

This story from Patient Opinion demonstrates how patient confidence and care are affected by the experience of poor organisation and communication in healthcare:

> My wife is due to have wrist surgery at ******** Hospital today. We met her consultant on Monday and were given an admission letter which said Ward ** would call us to give her an admission time. We were told to expect the call during Thursday. By 4pm yesterday we still had not heard anything so I tried to call the ward several times as mostly the number just rang out. When they eventually answered they said admission was normally 7.30am but that since we hadn't been given a time we would be called in the morning after the consultants had met to discuss the list for the day. We were told to expect the call after 8.30am. So when the phone rang around that time today I was somewhat surprised to be rudely told that my wife was meant to be in for surgery at 7.30 today. I explained exactly what we had been told and that the communication had been unhelpful and non-existent. The staff member went to speak to the consultant and seemed more contrite when asking me to bring my wife in asap. However on our arrival this same staff member proceeded to argue with me telling me they had called us 2 days ago and spoken to me when that hadn't been the case.
>
> I'm not stupid and know exactly what's happened when and I really object to being treated like we were in the wrong. Now we've arrived in day surgery they don't know if she's having an operation in the morning or afternoon and her notes aren't here. If we didn't know and trust her consultant, we'd be going home because the organisation and communication has been nothing but farcical.
>
> (www.patientopinion.org.uk)

Organisations, culture, communication and leadership

On qualification, you will be working in a healthcare organisation of some description. Organisations consist of groups of people who share a set of goals. The manner in which they operate could be construed as 'a social arrangement for the controlled performance of collective goals with a boundary controlling the relationships the organisation has with its environment' (Barr and Dowding, 2008, p. 156). In healthcare, the goal is to provide compassionate and effective care.

It is important that organisations maintain both a sense of the direction and the vision of the service to be provided and that they be cognisant of the mechanisms and processes that they will use to achieve these aims. Without this strategy, the ability to function effectively and compassionately will be compromised. In an ever-changing environment such as the health service, meeting this remit can be challenging, and as events from recent years have illustrated, this has not always been successfully achieved.

The failings by the Mid Staffordshire NHS Foundation Trust exemplify this perspective, whereby the lack of an informed and responsive understanding of the organisation resulted in dire consequences for patients. The subsequent investigations into performance by Francis (2013) levied a number of criticisms on the Trust. These included concerns about the culture, a target-driven focus, inadequate processes, poor management of care, poor practice not being addressed and a lack of compassion.

Clearly, there are lessons for all who work within the health setting. In the quest for improvement, it would seem sensible for employees to have a better understanding of how information is communicated and acted on. Indeed, there are now calls for organisations to collate the necessary information for them to understand the issues relating to quality and to respond accordingly (Berwick, 2013). Important actions in redressing such issues include more transparent and safe systems; better detection of problems; ensuring the patient voice is heard; better responses to poor practice; clear channels of accountability; staff training; and addressing low levels of motivation (Department of Health, 2015).

These can read as a list of actions to take and processes to be addressed, and by itself will not lead to a more communicative, compassionate and patient-focused service. Hence, the dual focus on improving quality of care, by reviewing actions required, and incorporating an understanding of the organisational culture (Francis, 2013; Department of Health, 2015). In order to be able to respond to this requisite, staff will need to have an understanding of the factors that impact organisational culture.

Organisational culture

Organisational culture relates to the practices and behaviours that are deemed to be the pattern or norm within the organisation. Interestingly, such behaviours and responses may not have direct association with the policies and procedures that are in place within the organisation. They may, for example, be dependent on individual reactions, specific to some services or endemic throughout the organisation. The nature of the response is important and of course only becomes problematic if the reactions emulated have negative correlations. However, even if the organisation is functioning well, the appreciation of what factors enable this is equally important.

Evidently, there is a lot of work to be done, however unpicking the elements contributing to the dynamics of culture in a meaningful way is potentially challenging. The Competing Values Framework offers a useful way of understanding the nature of organisational culture by providing a synopsis of the types of behaviour and issues that could occur (Cameron and Quinn, 2005). This model has deconstructed organisational behaviour into four prevailing cultures of hierarchical, adhocracy, market and clan.

Competing values framework

- hierarchical – a focus on bureaucracy and rules and regulations
- adhocracy – a flexible approach concerned with the ability to be creative and innovative
- market – an emphasis on external affairs, for example the measurement of organisational performance in relation to competitors
- clan – the sense of belonging and teamwork.

This structure can provide some understanding of where the organisation may tend to focus, and how an appreciation of this will be key to its performance. However, there is a sense that the area of clan culture is one area particularly attributable to being beneficial for both the organisation and the patient, and thus is especially important in the health environment (Carrillo, 2012; West et al., 2015).

Given this, an understanding of how well staff feel engaged with an organisation is pivotal to the quality of care provided and the organisation's standing, and one that strategic leaders need to be mindful of. There is a corresponding onus on staff to play their own part in understanding how they too can create such facilitative environments.

So what does this mean in terms of practice?

_____ CRITICAL THINKING EXERCISE 11.1 _____
REFLECTION POINT

- Consider an area where you have worked.
- How much focus do you feel was spent on each of the cultural perspectives identified in the competing values framework?

Once you have completed this, reflect on (1) what sort of behaviour was prevalent; and (2) what the consequences were for the team and the organisation in exercise 11.2.

_____ CRITICAL THINKING EXERCISE 11.2 _____
ORGANISATIONAL CULTURE

Culture	Clinical perspective
Hierarchical	How much attention was paid to ensuring rules were applied?
	Did you feel that this assisted or prevented your working?
Adhocracy	How open was the practice area to new ideas, or adapting ways of working?
Market	Did you know how well the service was performing?
	How did this compare to other similar practices outside of the service/organisation?
Clan	How well did the team function?
	What sort of leadership style was used?

The importance of self in leadership

As you progress on your nursing programme, the expectation that you will take more responsibility in clinical areas will become apparent. The assessment and feedback processes will have offered an indication of progress, but how clear are you in regard to understanding your leadership and management communication skills?

CRITICAL THINKING EXERCISE 11.3
LEADERSHIP AND YOU

How do you view leadership and management?

- instantly forgotten words
- not for me now
- something that more senior people do.

If you have answered yes to any of these, then you are not alone. Many student nurses would argue that they are too busy honing their clinical skills to worry about this. However, this outlook is problematic, and a lack of appreciation of the importance of leadership can potentially be difficult for both the individual and the organisation.

There is general agreement that nursing students are ill equipped for the transition to staff nurse, and that during their training they need to consider their progress in terms of building leadership and management skills. So when should this transition start? Nursing students at all levels will be exhibiting some form of leadership. The task for any individual rests with the need to acknowledge that they are already demonstrating leadership, and to explore the level of leadership they personally operate within. For example, how can one say that they will advocate for a patient without applying some leadership skills? Equally, when tasked with demonstrating the ability to manage a ward, it is not possible to do so without showing some authority and understanding of what needs to happen and managing the situation in hand.

Molly, our student midwife, describes her experience of leadership, co-ordination and teamwork.

Thus, far from being purely the remit of those who hold authority and power, leadership is already at play, and entails individuals building and developing such skills from the outset of their clinical placements. As such, understanding your current approaches to leadership is a starting point, and fundamental to building and honing such skills. So, what is leadership?

Student story 11.2: Molly and teamwork

Midway through the shift, the emergency buzzer goes off. You leave the woman you're looking after and run to it. Everyone is there. You need to portray confidence and control of the situation. During an emergency, it's easy to forget that there is a woman at the centre of it

(Continued)

(Continued)

all and, very likely, a terrified partner looking on. You need to give comfort and reassurance quickly, whilst a changing situation is going on around you. Communication with your team is also crucial: what's happening, what do we do, how do we do it, can someone pass me that, please? Sometimes, off to theatre we go; if the birth has already happened, this can leave behind a dad holding his brand new baby and imagining the worst possible outcome – he needs support too. After the event, that couple will pore over every detail and replay the scenario in their heads – so will you, in some cases! If they felt informed as to what was happening, and reassured by the way the team worked together, their memories of that experience are likely to be much more manageable for them.

Leadership

A leader can be conceived as someone who leads a group or an organisation to complete a task and motivates others to do the same. The term is frequently associated with particular types of communicative behaviour or skills that engage followers (see Table 11.1).

Table 11.1   Leadership behaviour

Good Communicator	Innovator	Visionary	Empathetic
Courageous	Persistent	Charismatic	Motivator
Trustworthy	Insightful	Decisive	Responsible

Leadership traits

- Trait theory: this explores the idea that characteristics of an individual will influence the ability to be a leader.
- Skills viewpoint: the skills perspective correlates with the development of specific capabilities that will enhance leadership abilities.
- Behaviour standpoint: focuses on the leadership response that individuals might have in managing a situation. (Yukl, 2012)

In general, it is the skills focus and behaviour standpoints that receive the most attention, and this is largely because of the possibilities of being able to improve performance. For instance, some perspectives equate leadership behaviour with four areas of being relationship focused – supporting others, dealing with the task, managing change processes, and networking (Yukl, 2012).

Other ideas focus on the response to managing a situation – see, for example, Table 11.2.

Table 11.2   Leadership style

Leadership style	Associated decision-making behaviour
Autocratic	Forthright, driven, can be task-focused
Democratic	Consultative, relationship building
Bureaucratic	Reliant on policies and procedure
Laissez Faire	Minimal input

Source: Lewin et al. (1939)

Individuals may prefer to use any one of these behaviours, however understanding your preferred default position will be helpful in unpicking how to manage situations.

Leadership ideology and skill sets transcend all organisations and thus are relevant to any company setting. However, a detailed health-focused appreciation of the skills needed is offered by the NHS Leadership Academy that has devised the Health Care Leadership Model (2013). This incorporates nine dimensions that are deemed important in the development of leadership, along with an outline of the activities that might be required in each section (see Table 11.3).

Table 11.3   Healthcare leadership model

Leading with care	Overseeing and looking after the team needs
Sharing the vision	Communicating the way forward
Engaging the team	Valuing the individual in the team
Evaluating information	Gathering the right information for improvement
Inspiring shared purpose	Showing commitment and being a role model
Holding to account	Supporting people to manage goals
Connecting our services	Understanding of interdisciplinary perspectives
Developing capability	Providing an environment conducive for personal and staff development
Influencing for results	Using interpersonal skills in order to build a collaborative workspace where contributions and concerns are recognised

Source: NHS Leadership Academy (2013)

This perspective is shared by the Kings Fund (2011) which argues that collaborative relationships and good communication are much more effective than autocratic, heroic leaders.

So what does this mean for you as a leader?

Consider the following situation – perhaps something similar has happened to you or someone that you know. Reflect on your communicative response.

CRITICAL THINKING EXERCISE 11.4
SCENARIO – THE 'TROUBLESOME' HCA

You have been asked to manage a bay of patients with an experienced healthcare assistant. She appears stressed and you hear her grumbling under her breath about the workload, and on a number of occasions she is very abrupt with you in front of others, including patients. You and other team members are finding this upsetting. Additionally, you note that on several occasions she does not complete the correct hand-washing procedures.

Would you:

- ignore it?
- step in and address the issues?
- negotiate with her?
- confront the issues?

 Visit the Values Exchange website at http://sagecomms.vxcommunity.com to develop your critical thinking skills and debate your thoughts and decisions.

First of all, there is the practical unpicking and understanding:

- What do you think the issues are?
- What management issues are important here?
- How might you resolve these?

Perhaps the first question you might ask yourself is: what are the techniques that I can learn so that I can practise them effectively and deal with such situations?

Clearly, it is important to address the situation, as there are potentially negative ramifications for both the patients and the team. However, the options for managing this are arguably less clear cut. The answers are not purely dependent on how proficient an individual is in achieving a task, but also reliant on how well they can analyse not only the situational dynamics but also their own personal tools and resources within such contexts.

Undoubtedly, there are some ideas, concepts and techniques that are useful, though they will have little merit without the inclusion of a key ingredient – understanding self. Indeed, the NHS Leadership Academy identifies personal qualities of self-awareness, self-confidence, self-knowledge, personal reflection, resilience and determination as key components in the development of leadership skills.

However, given the need for improvement in patient outcomes, and striving for a better healthcare organisational culture, one particular style seems especially pertinent, and comes in the shape of 'authentic leadership'. Further endorsement suggests that this particular style of working provides the necessary foundation on which leadership could be developed (Avolio and Gardner, 2005).

Authentic self and authentic leadership

Authentic leadership stems from a relationship-oriented perspective and is attributable to people who 'know who they are and what they believe and value, and act upon those values and beliefs while transparently interacting with others' (Avolio et al., 2004, p. 802).

As an aspiring leader, the notion of not only understanding yourself, but also having an appreciation of these skills in relation to the requirements of your followers, is salient. An authentic leadership approach appears to allow for both these perspectives. In particular, behaving authentically creates a supportive and collaborative setting where people feel they belong (Laschinger et al., 2012). Importantly, this not only positively affects the development of that individual, but also positively impacts on the personal development of followers (Avolio et al., 2009).

The benefits of authentic leadership

- improved quality of patient care
- reduction in staff sickness
- the work environment is perceived as supportive towards the individual
- improved teamwork
- employees feel able to discuss ideas and concerns
- increased creativity.

Components of authentic leadership

The concept of authenticity is associated with the four components of self-awareness, relational transparency, internalised moral perspectives and balanced processing (Walumbwa et al., 2008). Each of these elements is explored further.

Self-awareness

This relates to the ability to constantly review, renew and revise personal skills, in a bid to appreciate the changing and unchanging self. Reviewing behaviour in this manner provides the opportunity to explore a number of facets, including strengths, weaknesses, values and beliefs. The ultimate purpose of such actions is to increase the ability to engage and work with others.

The exploration of self also provides a means to appreciate how events have shaped an individual's perspective of the world, which is deemed to be key to developing and maintaining authenticity (Walumbwa et al., 2008). Fundamentally, it is about building an understanding of self and appreciating why you respond to situations in the manner that you do.

Once there is some appreciation of self, these lessons can provide a frame for building on self-leadership. Having this clarity will enable the opportunity to build on your understanding of self, appreciate the behaviour you normally use, and then decide if it is the correct response for the situation encountered. The ensuing insights enhance the opportunity to achieve, learn from failure and set goals for improving progress (Houghton et al., 2012).

Importantly, it needs to be remembered that whilst many nurses will appreciate the need to provide patient-focused care, this objective for achieving quality care also needs to incorporate authenticity. Arguably, this is a skill that can only be achieved through self-awareness and the appreciation of leadership (Waite et al., 2014).

Relational transparency

This aspect relates to being able to appropriately express authenticity of self, but doing so in a way that is salient to the circumstances involved (Avolio et al., 2009). This requires the ability to have a degree of honesty and openness but, at the same time, to also avoid inappropriate emotions (Walumbwa et al., 2008). Emotional intelligence, self-compassion and understanding the voice are useful standpoints for considering this authentic construct.

Emotional intelligence

We return to the concept of managing emotions described under the umbrella of emotional intelligence. Essentially, it can be viewed as a concept conceived as relating to specific skills, abilities and personality behaviours that have been learnt, which enable a person to distinguish their own emotions, as well as those of other people (Bulmer-Smith et al., 2009). They are able to explore situations, remain cognisant of their own personal characteristics, and use emotions, as a means to understand their feelings (Rankin, 2013).

Certainly, it seems that being able to effectively control and direct emotions provides the space and opportunity to see things differently. For example, in conflict situations, the ability to focus in this way provides an opportunity to understand matters from a new standpoint, and consider strategies that will enable the learning to be more positively framed. Approaching situations in this manner allows for opportunities to increase personal effectiveness. Given the range of emotions that nursing students and qualified staff experience in their daily work, it is suggested that an understanding of this concept is an important part of developing staff (Bulmer-Smith et al., 2009).

Self-compassion

This is a further example of the need to manage emotions. The expectation that nurses are compassionate is an implicit notion, but we can consider the delivery of compassionate care as comprising of two strands: first, instrumental *caring*, which centres around having the necessary skills to complete a task, and second, *expressive caring*, which focuses on the emotions (Davison and Williams, 2008). Neglecting the emotional element can lead to nurses being viewed as lacking compassion. The difficulty is that continuous exposure to events, and a lack of attention to their own personal needs, can cause nurses to dissociate from a patient, and only complete the task component. In order to avoid this, nurses must also spend some time caring for their own needs (see more on this in Chapter 12).

Self-compassion could be considered a mixture of mindfulness, self-kindness and wisdom that has benefits for both the individual and others (Reyes, 2012). It is an evolving process that grows alongside personal learning, and as such is directly linked to how you care for yourself and others.

The reference to wisdom is especially salient, and can be subdivided into three further areas. First, being able to self-appraise one's actions is an idea similar to emotional intelligence, in that understanding the benefits and deficits of the same thing is important. The second and third aspects of wisdom are being able to reflect and to have a non-judgemental attitude towards others. These perspectives are also featured within the overall concepts of authentic leadership. Thus, self-compassion can be seen to have direct links to the way that we can lead authentically.

So what steps can assist in growth of this area?   In the concept model for self-compassion, Reyes (2012) suggests the following strategies for building capability in this area:

- recognising you are not managing or becoming dissociated
- appreciating the need to change
- being kind to yourself and putting strategies in place to redress this.

Completion of these steps will increase individual positivity and the ability to relate to self and others.

These may seem obvious steps but, unfortunately, the need for self-compassion is often not appreciated by many nurses, and there is a tendency for them not to care for themselves. The obvious repercussions of failing to do so lie in nurses falling prey to stress and burnout and increased sickness rates. Aside from the effects on the nurse, there is growing evidence to indicate that nurses' wellbeing has a direct link to the quality of care that patients will receive, thus it is a factor that cannot be ignored.

Voice

Working and providing care within any organisation mean that you are part of the organisation and therefore also ostensibly part of creating the path or environment that encourages the discussion of issues, including those that are problematic in some way. The reality is that there may be some reluctance from staff to confront issues, and evidence indicates that nursing students and recently graduated nurses are especially weak in ensuring their perspectives are noted (Law and Chan, 2015). Some of the reasons for this lie with concern about how ideas might be received, along with the fear of negative responses from team members (Morrison and Milliken, 2003).

In some ways, the ability to speak up is dependent on the perceived safety of the setting, and is closely associated with how much followers feel able to voice opinions and concerns, and how they think the organisation might respond (Okuyama et al., 2014). Naturally, this is problematic, as a failure to speak out about their concerns will mean that issues are not addressed and patient care is compromised.

A key enabling factor is how an organisation reacts to hearing concerns. In response, a number of organisations have now provided listening opportunities to redress such anxieties. However, it is recognised that the actions of teams and individuals can also be an influencing factor on speaking-up behaviour, so the opportunities to change can also occur at a local level.

It is easy to appreciate how the individual perspective continually links back to the team and organisational experience, and the importance of having supportive facilitative processes is crucial. There is also an onus on individuals to consider what formal and informal support mechanisms are available to help them manage and learn from their emotional responses. This includes the 'need to keep a balanced and focused approach, along with the components of recognising situations when your personal resources may be drained' (NHS England, 2014, p. 7).

CRITICAL THINKING EXERCISE 11.5
RELATIONAL TRANSPARENCY – REFLECTIONS

How confident are you in speaking out about:

- poor patient care?
- the needs of other team members?
- your own needs?

What strategies do you use to manage your emotions at work? Remember the strategies from Part 1?

What mechanisms of support are available to you? Do you use these?

Moral perspective

This third authentic construct is steered by a person's own beliefs and standards, and correlates with a need for setting the standards and behaviours that the leader wants their followers to emulate.

The primary focus here is on appreciating and understanding personal values, and expressing these in a manner that others can see. The significance of this behaviour lies in the facilitative environment that can be created, allowing the values of trust and respect to thrive.

The importance of staff feeling safe enough to discuss concerns and ideas has already been mentioned, and creating the right environment is an important factor in allowing this to happen. Once staff are able to access a facilitative space, this will enable them to identify concerns, and allow the leader or organisation to respond to them. There are always elements of practice that can be improved, and as such this approach should be viewed as an ongoing opportunity to improve service provision.

An important feature of the creation of a clear moral standard is that of trust. The best approaches to achieving trust lie with the use of empowering and supportive leadership behaviours, including others in decision making and trying to ensure that the results are clearly managed (Wong and Cummings, 2009). For this to happen, leaders will need to ensure that their decisions also marry up with their moral perspectives (Laschinger et al., 2012). Such conduct may then be emulated by followers, and thus have the potential to positively affect not only the individual but also the team and the organisation.

In practice, nursing students may find this challenging, as trying to raise concerns or suggest ideas can conflict with the perceived need to be compliant (Jack and Wibberley, 2014). Nonetheless, developing skills where individuals are seen to be engaging and honest with others ultimately helps with how well followers will engage and affects how the organisation itself is perceived (Leroy et al., 2012).

CRITICAL THINKING EXERCISE 11.6
VALUES

- What values are important to you?
- How do you demonstrate these at work?
- How have you responded when these have been breached?
- Think of someone who is able to maintain his or her moral perspective. Consider what this looks like and how it feels.

Balanced processing

This fourth and final construct of authentic leadership is concerned with the ability to process and analyse information. Part of this process includes the expectation that individuals will be able to ask for opinions on their behaviour, and also able to cope with the answers, even if these responses might challenge their perspective (Waite et al., 2014). The remit also sees the ability to capture both negative and positive experiences and unpick these as a further learning point.

Perhaps the best opportunity to complete this lies with appreciating the need for reflection and mindfulness, both of which have been mentioned in relation to other aspects in previous chapters. However, we need to also consider this in terms of leadership and how this can be incorporated as part of balanced processing.

Being mindful calls for the need to be present and self-aware, whilst at the same time acting as an observer, examining the body response to situations, but not getting caught up in emotions (Khong, 2011). Achieving this will require practice, however the benefits will be reaped when the individual is able to capture their own response but also allow for understanding the emotion of another (White, 2014).

We should also be cognisant of the fact that lack of mindfulness is reported to correlate with poor patient care and experience (Wong et al., 2013); and mindfulness is suggested as an aspect that can be included as one of the personal expectations of management of self (NHS England, 2014).

Critical debate 11.1

Leadership is only for those who want to climb the career ladder. Ordinary nurses and mid-wives don't need to be leaders. Discuss.

Conclusion

This chapter has considered the communicative behaviours in leadership and management. Leadership is often considered irrelevant to newly qualified nurses and midwives but it is expected and the transition period can be particularly testing. The chapter explored the notion of organisations and their cultures and went on to examine the concept, behaviours and communicative elements of leadership. Applying the concepts from the competing values framework and using the four authentic leadership constructs are useful strategies on which to build the necessary skills for creating an authentic organisational culture. As with other aspects of communication, the ability to be self-aware and self-compassionate enhances leadership capacity.

Further suggested activity

Go to www.kingsfund.org.uk/leadership to explore some of the thinking around how leadership can be developed across all levels in healthcare. Read the blogs.

Sign yourself up for emails from Roy Lilley at www.nhsmanagers.net

Also see the Foundation of Nursing Leadership at www.nursingleadership.org.uk/

To access further resources related to this chapter, visit the Values Exchange website at http:// sagecomms.vxcommunity.com

References

Avolio, B.J. and Gardner, W.L. (2005) 'Authentic leadership development: getting to the root of positive forms of leadership', *The Leadership Quarterly*, 16(3): 315–38.

Avolio, B.J., Gardner, W.L., Walumbwa, F.O., Luthans, F., and May, D.R. (2004) 'Unlocking the mask: a look at the process by which authentic leaders impact follower attitudes and behaviors', *Leadership Quarterly*, 15: 801–23.

Avolio, B.J., Walumbwa, F.O. and Weber, T.J. (2009) 'Leadership: current theories, research, and future directions', *Annual Review of Psychology*, 60: 421–49.

Barr, J. and Dowding, L. (2008) *Leadership in Health Care*. London: Sage.

Berwick, D. (2013) *A Promise to Learn: A Commitment to Act – Improving the Safety of Patients in England*. London: Department of Health.

Bulmer Smith, K., Profetto-McGrath, J. and Cummings G.G. (2009) 'Emotional intelligence and nursing: an integrative literature review', *International Journal of Nursing Studies*, 46(12): 1624–36.

Cameron, K.S. and Quinn, R.E. (2005) *Diagnosing and Changing Organizational Culture: Based on the Competing Values Framework*. Chichester: John Wiley & Sons.

Carrillo, R.A. (2012) 'Relationship-based safety moving beyond culture and behavior', *Professional Safety*, 57(12): 35–45.

Davison, N. and Williams, K. (2008) 'Compassion in nursing, 1: defining, identifying and measuring this essential quality', *Nursing Times*, 105(36): 16–18.

Department of Health (2015) *Culture Change in the NHS: Applying the Lessons of the Francis Inquiries*. London: HMSO.

Francis, R. (2013) *Report of the Mid Staffordshire NHS Foundation Trust Public Inquiry*. London: The Stationery Office.

Houghton, J.D., Wu, J., Godwin, J.L., Neck, C.P. and Manz, C.C. (2012) 'Effective stress management: a model of emotional intelligence, self-leadership, and student stress coping', *Journal of Management Education*, 36(2): 220–38.

Jack, K. and Wibberley, C. (2014) 'The meaning of emotion work to student nurses: a Heideggerian analysis', *International Journal of Nursing Studies*, 51(6): 900–7.

Kings Fund (2011) *No More Heroes*. Available at: www.kingsfund.org.uk/sites/files/kf/future-of-leadership-and-management-nhs-may-2011-kings-fund (accessed 7 November 2012).

Khong, B.S.L. (2011) 'Mindfulness: a way of cultivating deep respect for emotions', *Mindfulness*, 2(1): 27–32.

Laschinger, H.K.S., Wong, C.A. and Grau, A.L. (2012) 'The influence of authentic leadership on newly graduated nurses' experiences of workplace bullying, burnout and retention outcomes: a cross-sectional study', *International Journal of Nursing Studies*, 49(10): 1266–76.

Law, B.Y. and Chan, E.A. (2015) 'The experience of learning to speak up: a narrative inquiry on newly graduated registered nurses', *Journal of Clinical Nursing*, 24(13–14): 1837–48.

Leroy, H., Palanski, M. E. and Simons, T. (2012) *Authentic Leadership and Behavioral Integrity as Drivers of Follower Commitment and Performance* [electronic version]. Available at: http://scholarship.sha.cornell.edu/articles/723 (accessed 10 May 2016).

Lewin, K., Llippit, R. and White, R.K. (1939) 'Patterns of aggressive behavior in experimentally created social climates', *Journal of Social Psychology*, 10: 271–301.

Morrison, E.W. and Milliken, F.J. (2003) 'Speaking up, remaining silent: the dynamics of voice and silence in organizations', *Journal of Management Studies*, 40(6): 1353–8.

NHS England (2014) 'Building and strengthening leadership: leading with compassion', November. London: NHS England. Available at: www.england.nhs.uk/wp-content/uploads/2014/12/london-nursing-accessible.pdf (accessed 16 April 2016).

NHS Leadership Academy (2013) *Healthcare Leadership Model*. Available at: www.leadershipacademy.nhs.uk/resources/healthcare-leadership-model/ (accessed 10 May 2016).

Okuyama, A., Wagner, C. and Bijnen, B. (2014) 'Speaking up for patient safety by hospital-based health care professionals: a literature review', *BMC Health Services Research*, 14(1): 61.

Rankin, B. (2013) 'Emotional intelligence: enhancing values-based practice and compassionate care in nursing', *Journal of Advanced Nursing*, 69(12): 2717–25.

Reyes, D. (2012) 'Self-compassion: a concept analysis', *Journal of Holistic Nursing*, 30(2): 81–9.

Waite, R., McKinney, N., Smith-Glasgow, M.E. and Meloy, F.A. (2014) 'The embodiment of authentic leadership', *Journal of Professional Nursing*, 30(4): 282–291.

Walumbwa, F.O., Avolio, B.J., Gardner, W.L., Wernsing, T.S. and Peterson, S.J. (2008) 'Authentic leadership: development and validation of a theory-based measure', *Journal of Management*, 34(1): 89–126.

West, M., Armit, K., Loewenthal, L., Eckert, R., West, T. and Lee, A., (2015) *Leadership and Leadership Development in Healthcare: The Evidence Base*. London: The King's Fund. Available at: www.kingsfund.org.uk/sites/files/kf/field/field_publication_file/leadership-leadership-develop ment-health-care-feb-2015.pdf (accessed 16 April 2016).

White, L. (2014) 'Mindfulness in nursing: an evolutionary concept analysis', *Journal of Advanced Nursing*, 70(2): 282–94.

Wong, C.A., Cummings, G. and Ducharme, L. (2013) 'The relationship between nursing leadership and patient outcomes: a systematic review update', *Journal of Nursing Management*, 21(5): 709–24.

Wong, G. and Cummings, G. (2009) 'The influence of authentic leadership behaviors on trust and work outcomes of health care staff ', *Journal of Leadership Studies*, 3 (2): 6–23.

Yukl, G. (2012) 'Effective leadership behavior: what we know and what questions need more attention', *The Academy of Management Perspectives*, 26(4): 66–85.

12

Maintaining Positive Values in Communication and Caring for Self and Others

Armin Luthi and Iris Gault

• • • • • • • • • • • Learning Objectives • • • • • • • • • • •

By the end of this chapter, you will have developed an understanding of:

- the emotional challenges of transitioning to qualified nurse status
- how to sustain and enhance ethical and compassionate communication in difficult circumstances
- learning from the past.

 Don't forget to visit the Values Exchange website at http://sagecomms.vxcommunity.com for extra practice and revision activities.

• •

Introduction

In this chapter, we are going to look at how to help you consolidate and sustain the skills, knowledge and insight you have developed over the duration of completing this book. We are also going to focus on how you can do this during the transition period you make as you adapt from being a student to a qualified nurse. Being in full-time employment and offering your 'labour' is a very different experience to being a student nurse, and this massive change (with all its considerations, meanings and implications for your 'emotional labour') will be a core feature throughout this chapter. Therefore, it examines the challenges of facing your first post as a professional and goes on to look at strategies to overcome anxiety and help maintain your ability to communicate compassionately despite difficult circumstances. It concludes by returning to some of the issues raised by inquiries into poor communication and considers what we can learn from these.

Student story 12.1: Return to Josh

Josh is a third-year mental health nursing student. He is now 24 and approaching the end of his course. Josh had worked as a healthcare assistant in a mental health forensic unit prior to entering nurse education. When Josh started his course, he is a bit ashamed to say that he thought he already knew most of what he needed to know about communicating with others. Over the past two and a half years, he has realised how much he had to learn. However, he buckled down and is now rated as having very good communication skills in practice. His mentor in practice (Josh was sponsored by his Trust to do his training and his Trust mentor told him that his communication skills needed addressing) now feels that Josh will be a very effective mental health nurse.

It's looking likely that he will take up his first post in one of the mental health forensic wards. He's looking forward to it but he is wondering how he can make sure he retains and develops his enthusiasm. He's also thinking about how he's going to work with some of the other nurses and healthcare assistants who seem a bit jaded and less caring.

Visit the Values Exchange website at http://sagecomms.vxcommunity.com for a broader discussion on Josh's story.

Student story 12.2: Return to Molly

Molly is a third-year midwifery student. The end of her course is very close and she is looking forward to being a newly qualified midwife. She loves the work but it is intense and she is also slightly apprehensive about being a fully fledged professional without the student support systems. The mothers seem to like Molly; feedback has indicated that they find her to be supportive and trustworthy. Molly has high standards for herself and is determined to maintain her competence and her approachable manner. However, she has noticed that some of the qualified midwives seem to have become less service user-focused as time goes on. They are not unpleasant to the mothers but they don't really see them as individuals and seem to just want to get through the shift. Molly is sure she'll never be like that, but wonders how she will manage to retain her enthusiasm when work is so busy.

Visit the Values Exchange website at http://sagecomms.vxcommunity.com for a broader discussion on Molly's story.

The emotional challenges of transitioning to qualified nurse status

Why are we so focused on this? Whilst it is hard to formalise and describe this transition, we know it is incredibly challenging. So, whilst it is very much an experiential 'lived through' process, it is also essential that you are prepared for it. We have already talked a lot about the concept of 'change' and its many complications and the role of personal awareness and understanding in managing it, and those same principles apply here. I am sure, right now, at this moment in time, nearing the end of your training, you are probably very eager to get to grips with the transition, in the expectation that it will be very similar to all the other changes and transitions you have made through years 1 to 3 of your training. However, you need to be mindful that there will be some key differences.

CRITICAL THINKING EXERCISE 12.1
FACING THE TRANSITION

At the moment, you will have been thinking about finishing your course and getting your qualification. Try to think back over your experience of training. What is the biggest change that you can see in yourself? And how did it come about? Spend about 10 minutes reflecting on this, and write down your reflections:

- How did this change come about? Was it very quick? Or was it more gradual?
- Did you notice this change in yourself or did other people point it out to you?
- How did it feel to recognise that you had changed? Try and identify both the positives and the negatives of this experience.

'Making the transition from student to qualified nurse is a stressful experience. Literature on the issue indicates this is not confined to the UK but transcends international boundaries' (Whitehead, 2011, p. 20). There are a number of key changes that happen on qualification. As a student, you were protected in many ways from the realities of clinical work, not least because you were never fully responsible for your clients. There was also the impermanence of your placements, and the ongoing focus on you and your personal and professional development. In addition, as a student, you were also given the full weight of support from both your university and your mentor.

However, with the transition, this all stops abruptly and, whilst you might still see yourself (to some degree) as a novice, the people around you will not. They will see you as a fully accountable practitioner who is completely clinically responsible for every decision and action undertaken on duty, and no matter how committed, competent and enthusiastic you might be as a student, this is a very different position in which to find yourself. The NMC itself recognises this and has developed the process of preceptorship to enhance and consolidate the newly qualified nurse's position as they evolve into their new role and identity, and in this chapter we want to support this process and offer a way and a means for you to prepare yourself for what can be a challenging and demanding experience (Edwards et al., 2011).

As you might expect, and in keeping with the rest of the book, our starting point, for this chapter, is ourselves. How do you see the transition applying to you? Do you expect things to run smoothly? Or do you think that there might be some hurdles? Do you feel secure and confident in yourself? Or are you feeling any anxiety? And if you are experiencing anxiety, what are you feeling that anxiety about?

CRITICAL THINKING EXERCISE 12.2
IMAGINE IT'S THE FIRST DAY IN YOUR FIRST JOB AS A QUALIFIED NURSE...

- How are you feeling?
- Why?

- What's going through your mind?
- What are you saying to yourself?
- Why?
- What do you notice about your body?
- Why?
- How have you prepared yourself?
- Why?

Spend 5–10 minutes exploring this scenario and write your answers down.

- What do you think are likely to be the biggest challenges facing you on this first day of work?
- And how do you plan to manage them?

Core reminder 1: Always remember the impact that anxiety can have on your thinking processes and the impact of fight, flight or freeze.

- Which of the above reactions happened to you in your hypothetical first-day scenario?

Sustaining and enhancing ethical and compassionate communication in difficult circumstances

Impact of anxiety (emotional mind) on decision making

The stressful experience of coping with the experience of being a qualified nurse is not a new phenomenon. Kramer (1974) identified the reality shock that confronted the newly registered nurse and how it contributed to some leaving the profession. Edwards et al. (2011) note that reality shock is still with us today, although Darvill et al. (2014) suggest this is more likely in acute, ward-based settings (often the first destination for the recently qualified). Whereas there is a responsibility for employers and educational institutions to adequately prepare students, there are some actions you can take yourself.

The first thing to be mindful of is anxiety. As noted in Chapter 2, we are all naturally anxious creatures (by nature and by biology), and because we are designed to be this way, anxiety is a natural and purposeful process rather than something that is alien, flawed or abnormal. Anxiety's key function is to help us survive in a dangerous and difficult world. As a survival strategy, anxiety is based on exactly the same processes as those we apply in nursing practice: assessment, identification and implementation. Remember that nursing is a problem-solving profession and, in this way, it is no different from the way anxiety operates in our minds: anxiety is designed to help us recognise and then solve a problem. Always remember that anxiety is actually a helpful thing and so it must not be avoided, ignored or denied.

However, anxiety needs to be kept in perspective, as we have to remember how easily we can be overwhelmed by it and lose the ability to problem solve. Our minds work on both an emotional and a logical level and these respective 'wires' sometimes get crossed, especially when we are tired, stressed, angry or hungry. You are likely to be very stressed in your first days as a qualified nurse, so be prepared!

_____   **CRITICAL THINKING EXERCISE 12.3**   _____
MOOD DIARY

Core reminder 2: Keep mood and thought diaries to help you identify, recognise and manage your particular thinking styles ... stay mindful! Be aware of when you are tired, stressed, angry, hungry or thirsty, and don't avoid or deny these states of mind or body.

Remember that if we don't *keep* reflecting on our anxieties, they can quickly go out of control ... and very easily. And then we fall into the trap of reacting to all our cognitive biases, conditional beliefs and schema, losing any sense of perspective or context and catastrophising everything.

Core reminder 3: We are all at constant risk of getting overwhelmed with anxiety, so stay mindful.

_____   **CRITICAL THINKING EXERCISE 12.4**   _____
IDENTIFY YOUR RESPONSE TO STRESS

Think back to a stressful experience that you had on placement ... what happened?

- What was the SITUATION?
- What EMOTIONS did you feel?
- What were you telling yourself (THOUGHTS)?
- What did you do (BEHAVIOUR)?

And, on reflection, what did you find out about yourself? How did your emotional mind react? And which of the many cognitive biases, conditional beliefs and schema did you find flooding your mind? What happened to your logical mind? Was it able to stay present with you? Or was it lost? Forgotten about? Or still there but ignored? And what did you do? *Fight? Flight? Freeze?* It is important that you stay very familiar with your anxiety response styles, as they are likely to crop up (*a lot*) during your transition/preceptorship phase, and unless you can recognise these, you will not be able to manage them.

Looking after yourself: the value and cost of emotional labour

Looking after oneself is key to anxiety management. As a student, I am sure that you were well supported through all your stressful experiences and were encouraged to reflect and learn from them (i.e. compassionate and emotionally fluent practice). You also had the framework of your university in place for you with a prevailing culture of tolerance and compassion. However, as we have seen from the example of Stafford Hospital, this support is unfortunately not guaranteed in clinical practice, and once you qualify this is something that you will need to manage yourself.

Msiska et al. (2014) studied student nurses in Malawi, working in stressful environments, caring for patients with HIV and AIDs. They concluded that those who were less able to attend to their own emotional needs were most at risk of developing non-compassionate attitudes towards and communication with their patients. Emotional exhaustion can lead to burnout and moral disengagement. Nursing care is incredibly hard work, but in many parts of the health services this seems taken for granted. Campbell (2015) notes that despite the pledge to provide adequate numbers of nurses to ensure safe patient care in the wake of reports into poor care, financial concerns seem to mean that this pledge has not been delivered. Organisations might talk about valuing nursing staff, but in practice put them in environments of unreasonable stress and demand, with little support. This may be further compounded by nursing cultures which assume that open and reflective dialogue about these emotional demands and stressors indicates character weakness rather than emotional intelligence (Townsend, 2012).

You may indeed already have experienced working in a placement area in which the prevailing culture was not supportive of emotionally intelligent reflective practice. The demands created by staff shortages, clinical pressure and waiting times and lists can compromise this, and compassion gets lost as a result. Nursing defines its role in terms of offering care, but this cannot just be assumed. Being able to endlessly offer care, no matter the demands and stresses laid on us, is not possible. We want to help you identify when this is happening to ensure that you do not become immersed in it, as it can be overwhelming.

Throughout the book, we have looked at how important it is to retain a sense of balance and perspective whilst working as a nurse, and we have seen how necessary it is for us to separate out our personal from our professional selves whilst delivering nursing care. We call this 'emotional labour', and it can be a controversial subject as some people see it vocationally (i.e. you offer it as a personal quality and it is your personal responsibility to keep offering it), and some as a professional learned process (that needs training, support and supervision to be sustained) (Gray and Smith, 2009). You will no doubt have seen and heard people say that nursing has 'changed' and that since it started to become an academic professional subject, it has 'lost the ability to care' for its clients (Goodman, 2015). However, evidence clearly indicates the fallacy of this vocational approach, as without the structure of an academic and professional framework (and the support mechanisms it offers) nurses may become overwhelmed and potentially lose their ability to care (Sawbridge and Hewison, 2011).

Subordination of nursing work

Confident professionalism is a factor in maintaining a compassionate attitude. In the midst of this vocation versus profession debate, healthcare is becoming increasingly consumer/customer-focused, and clients have the right to be highly critical of the quality of healthcare per se. However, the bulk of criticisms tend to be against nurses, and we need to be mindful that some of these criticisms are based on (vocationally focused) expectations of nursing care that originate in outdated and sexist stereotypes, rather than reflect the realities and pressures faced in contemporary nursing. In vocational terms, traditionally nursing was always to be a 'female exercise' as care was seen to be 'women's work'. Historically, this care was seen as inferior to the professional scientism of the (male) medical profession and, whilst social attitudes may have changed, Goodman (2015) states that it this continuing sexism which argues against nursing becoming an academic profession today: 'Or it could be seen as just a manifestation of the devaluing of nursing by society because nursing is care work, care is women's work and society does not value women's work' (Goodman and Ley, 2012, p. 39). For instance, in the *Meet the Fockers* films, one of the ongoing jokes at Ben Stiller's expense is the fact that, as a man, he has chosen nursing as a career (unlike his character's rival, the virile and competent Owen Wilson, who is a doctor).

We need to think about the impact of this subordination and how it might impair your professional practice. Hollinrake (2013) defines care as a social relational exercise, basic to the preservation of human life, entailing an interdependence and a vulnerability that are heavily influenced by individual, social, cultural and economic factors. Nursing can only function if its relationships are effective. However, in the utilisation of 'emotional labour', other factors need consideration, and these are often lost in the nursing process. Gabe (2013) argues that this situation is evidentially prevalent in clinical practice and that there is a need for other healthcare professions to strive for a more equal workplace situation.

Learning from the past

Understanding ourselves, our anxiety responses and the process of moral disengagement helps to enable us to identify and avoid negative communication, even within difficult circumstances. Emotional labour (EL) is described as the induction or suppression of feeling in order to sustain an outward persona that induces an emotion in others. In nursing, this kind of labour is controlled by employers and can be seen as a commodity that has an exchange value, even though it draws on a deep sense of self that is integral to the individual (Gray and Smith, 2009; Hochschild, 2012). Hochschild argues that people are socialised into learning the accepted 'feeling rules' that underpin socio-cultural expectations (i.e. be polite to relatives and betters, etc.). These are moral social values that act as constraints for the display of emotions (dependent on the situation etc.). This is 'emotion work', involving social acting (e.g. one might well cry at a funeral even though one does not feel sad, because one is expected to).

Because it is both so complex, so intrinsic to human relationships and also a commodity, she divides it into: surface acting – pretence as per 'the customer is always right' ('laughing politely' etc.), like flight attendants or bar staff – and deep acting – drawing on emotional memories in order to create feelings that are real and mirror others (empathy), like nurses.

How do you see your emotional labour and how much do you think 'being professional' is associated with being skilled at masking your true feelings? Hochschild (2012) argues that private emotion (deep acting) is exploited in the workplace, as it is transmuted into emotional labour. When this happens, staff are trained in the expression of appropriate emotions, in order to have the right 'state of mind' for the job, repressing or denying real feelings in the process, generally through the process of developing a therapeutic mindset, somewhat in the way that we have been showing you in this book. However, Smith (2012) says that nurses also offer their emotions as a 'gift', not as 'work', because the type of work that nurses do is far more complex, personally challenging and responsible than customer sales, for instance, and because of this, and because of the extreme vulnerability of our clients, we are held, as nurses, to be accountable for the quality of that gift of care. But when this gift is de-valued, unsupported and not allowed to be sustainable, nurses are likely to burn out and morally disengage from the whole process of care.

The process of moral disengagement is the culminating process of burnout. Goodman (2015) uses Bandura (1963) and Zimbardo (2004) to show how nurses morally disengage from professional and ethical practice. The extract in Patient story 12.1, taken from Patient Opinion, indicates how contrasting the experience of maternity care can be.

Patient story 12.1: An 'awful experience' versus a 'first-class experience'

I am so disappointed with the maternity department at ***** ***** Hospital. My daughter had a horrendous experience and I am appalled that this hospital is at third world level. The department is short staffed and this led to staff being rude, unhelpful and uncaring. When you are unable to move because of a spinal and a difficult birth, you should expect a healthcare assistant to be willing to change your baby for you. Not to get a sour response.

The receptionists are rude and unhelpful. Some nurses are rude and jobs worth, I genuinely think one in particular has become complacent and seems to be anti visitors. We felt so unwelcome. The whole negative experience has marred my daughter giving birth to a beautiful baby. This should have been a positive and happy experience. Thank goodness for ******** Hospital for being so different and lovely.

Yet, another experience at another unit, within the same time span, produced a very different outcome:

My wife arrived at the maternity ward fully dilated at 8.37am on Thursday 11th Feb: we were immediately taken to the birthing ward where 2 midwifes, one a trainee, quickly and professionally assessed my wife whilst making her comfortable – at 8.59 my beautiful baby daughter was born. The staff were exceptional not just for my wife but also myself. Their professional, knowledgeable and caring attitude helped tremendously in a traumatic situation when moved upstairs to the maternity ward room 1 across from reception. The fantastic service continued whilst on the ward.

****** hospital and the NHS in general should be proud of their midwives: all the support teams and doctors were fantastic and it made an amazing time for us even more amazing. Thank you to all involved especially from ******* and baby ******xxxx.

(www.patientopinion.org, 2016)

How do professionals disengage?

Process of moral disengagement

- They will reconstruct conduct, explaining their actions in minimalist and helpless terms, such as 'It is the best thing to do in the circumstances, so our only option'.
- They will displace responsibility, explaining their actions in minimalist and helpless terms, such as 'I'm just a nurse and I follow orders'.
- They will disregard injurious consequences, explaining their actions in minimalist and helpless terms, such as 'I will ignore or dismiss the likely results'.
- They will dehumanise or blame the client, explaining their actions in minimalist and helpless terms, such as 'They will get violent if we don't do this', 'They are drug users so what do they expect?'. (Zimbardo, 2004)

CRITICAL THINKING EXERCISE 12.5
MORAL DISENGAGEMENT

Have you seen examples of this type of moral disengagement:

- in yourself?
- in other nurses?

What did you do about it?

 Visit the Values Exchange website at http://sagecomms.vxcommunity.com to develop your critical thinking skills and debate your thoughts and decisions.

Sawbridge and Hewison (2011) assert that both individuals and organisations should understand and act to minimise the potential for moral disengagement in the healthcare workplace. At the start of this book, we talked about the Stafford nurses, and now we return to them. In Stafford, some people found themselves with their emotional intelligence so compromised by the prevailing organisational culture that they exhausted their capacity to offer their emotional labour and became morally disengaged instead. The Francis Report (2013) clearly described nursing staff who felt unsupported and became morally disengaged, resulting in poor care and uncompassionate communication with their patients. We have to face the possibility that this could happen to any one of us working in nursing care. Right now, as you prepare to qualify, you are especially vulnerable to this. However, understanding your emotions and utilising effective supervision can help you avoid falling into this trap. Use the skills and exercises given to you in this book.

Be self-aware

- Be self-aware and reflective.
- Be mindful of the impact of your work environment.
- Be mindful of its prevailing culture: is it professional, offering support, supervision and reflection time? With a democratic equalitarianism between all healthcare professionals?
- Or is it vocational, offering little support but expecting self-sacrifice, task-driven rituals and subordination to other professionals?
- And, if it is the latter, you will need to assert your right to getting support and supervision, as no one will do this for you.

Seek supervision and support

In this chapter, we have highlighted how long-standing and wider socio-cultural stereotypes can feel as though they de-value the nursing profession, falling back on old sexist ideas about the vocational nature of nursing care. Goodman (2015) argues that nurses will only defeat these stereotypes through becoming as politically assertive as other professionals and demanding the same level of continuing professional development supervision and support as received by other healthcare professionals.

Ask for clinical supervision to help you reflect on your work. Preceptorship schemes run in many (and should in all) healthcare organisations (see www.nhsemployers.org).

Whilst we remained trapped by old values about vocation and personal sacrifice, nurses will never be able to practise in such a way as to allow us to deeply act without loss of a private self because it is impossible to do this without sufficient support and supervision, and without the professional confidence to demand adequate resources without feeling guilty. There is recognition that the combination of an emotionally challenging job and punishing working practices can take a heavy toll on nurses and midwives, and various models of clinical supervision can be utilised. The Kings Fund evaluated Schwartz Centre Rounds. These rounds allow for an inter-professional space to discuss, reflect on and acknowledge the emotional labour of particular cases. This was a small pilot but Goodrich (2011) observed that Schwartz Centre Rounds appear to have benefits, and she suggests that similar interventions could be helpful in managing the emotional challenges of healthcare work. Wallbank and Preece (2010) noted that self-reported burnout decreased by 36% and stress generally by 59% when a system of clinical supervision was introduced in a health visiting service. As Sawbridge and Hewison (2011) note, these insights and interventions are not new. We know that working in healthcare is stressful; we know that stress can overwhelm and lead to moral disengagement and uncompassionate behaviour. Sawbridge and Hewison (2011) point out that we can learn from organisations such as the Samaritans where structured support is offered and is taken up. Townsend (2012), too, stresses that understanding the factors that influence the healthcare environment and our behaviour within that environment is essential in creating a healthy workplace that can provide compassionate and safe care: 'Treating all members of the healthcare team with respect leads to collaboration, open communication, and teamwork and promotes delivery of the high-quality care we all strive for' (2012, p. 15).

In Student story 12.3, one of our students tells the story of coping as a newly qualified midwife: the fast pace, the stress and also the importance of communicating with parents at this time in their lives.

Student story 12.3: A day in the life of Molly as a newly qualified midwife

A few months into your first job as a midwife, you are working on a busy delivery suite.

At any given time, you can have a number of situations going on that require you to be a swan: calm and unfussed to look at, but paddling furiously under the water! You walk into a room for the first time and have very little idea what to expect. You don't know how long you've got to build up a rapport with a woman and her family, whilst you care for them during, arguably, the most intense and unknown experience of their lives so far. You have to read situations carefully; throughout labour, most women's needs will change, sometimes needing you to talk them through, other times needing silence. You also have to balance all this with unending reams of paperwork! Women will say years down the line that they still remember their birth and, often, their midwife; you don't want that to be for the wrong reasons!

This excerpt demonstrates not only the challenge of remaining compassionate, competent and communicative, but also the satisfaction of working with people.

Critical debate 12.1

Is burnout inevitable? Can it really be prevented? Can we maintain the enthusiasm described above?

Conclusion

This chapter addresses one of the most difficult challenges for a nurse or midwife: how to maintain and sustain the enthusiasm and compassionate attitudes that drew them into healthcare in the first place. Inquiries and scandals of poor care tend to draw media attention rather than the areas where healthcare workers are getting it right, in continuing to provide compassionate care and helpful communication. Recognition and analysis of emotional labour and the psychological process that can lead to burnout or moral disengagement are essential in order to maintain and sustain compassionate practice. Confronting and acknowledging emotion as opposed to covering it up allows professionals to understand and deal with their work. The transition in the first few months will be challenging but newly qualified nurses have the right to demand (assertively, not aggressively) supervision and preceptorship, as in any profession. The need for this clinical supervision is recognised nationally and internationally, to support nurses and provide patients with safe and supportive care.

References

Bandura, A. (1963) 'Behavior theory and indemnificatory learning', *American Journal of Orthopsychiatry,* 33: 591–601.

Campbell, D. (2015) 'NHS "backtracking" on ward nurse numbers introduced after Mid Staffs', *The Guardian*, 13 October. Available at: www.theguardian.com/society/2015/oct/13/nhs-backtracking-on-ward-nurse-numbers-introduced-after-mid-staffs (accessed 16 April 2016).

Darvill, A.L., Fallon, D.M. and Livesley, J. (2014) 'A different world: the transition experiences of newly qualified children's nurses taking up first destination posts within children's community nursing teams in England', *Issues in Comprehensive Pediatric Nursing*, 37(1): 6–24.

Edwards, E., Hawkins, C., Carrier, J. and Rees, C. (2011) 'Effectiveness of strategies and interventions that aim to assist the transition from student to newly qualified nurse', *JBI Library of Systematic Reviews*, 9(53): 2215–23.

Francis, R. (2013) *Report of the Mid Staffordshire NHS Foundation Trust Public Inquiry*. London: The Stationery Office.

Gabe, J. (2013) 'Challenging the power of the medical profession', in J. Estermann, J. Page and U. Streckeisen (eds), *Alte und Neue Gesundheitsberufe* [Old and New Health Professions]. Zurich: LIT Verlag. pp. 20–36.

Goodman, B. (2015) 'Why do nurses behave as they do?', 20 February. Available at: www.bennygoodman.co.uk/why-do-nurses-behave-as-they-do/

Goodman, B. and Ley T. (2012) *Psychology and Sociology for Nurses* London: Sage

Goodrich, J. (2011) *Schwartz Center Rounds: Evaluation of UK Pilots*. London: Kings Fund.

Gray, B. and Smith, P. (2009) 'Emotional labour and the clinical settings of nursing care: the perspectives of nurses in East London', *Nurse Education in Practice*, 9(4): 253–61.

Hochschild, A.R. (2012) *The Managed Heart: Commercialization of Human Feeling*. Berkeley, CA: University of California Press.

13

Communication Theory, Reflective and Ethical Practice in the 'Swampy Lowlands'

Iris Gault

• • • • • • • • • • • Learning Objectives • • • • • • • • • • • •

By the end of this chapter, you will have developed an understanding of:

- the importance of communication theory
- communication, reflective and ethical practice
- communication theory that informs and enables reflection on ethical practice in healthcare.

 Don't forget to visit the Values Exchange website at http://sagecomms.vxcommunity.com for extra practice and revision activities.

• •

Introduction

This final chapter points the reader to more advanced understandings of communication theory and its relationship with ethical practice. Modern healthcare with advanced technology can be wonderfully effective yet failures of care still persist. Where these problems arise, they can often be traced back to difficulties with human communicative interaction. Donald Schön (1983, p. 3) coined the phrase, the 'swampy lowlands' of practice, where technical competence does not provide an answer to the complicated reality of life. Despite technical progress, the world of healthcare is challenging and it is a professional responsibility to practise competently and ethically. This includes the ability to communicate compassionately and effectively. Therefore, in this final chapter we suggest that students approaching qualification consider how they may develop a more in-depth, theoretical and reflective appreciation of their communicative practice.

At undergraduate level, the focus is on learning how to communicate well with patients and other professionals, informed by appropriate knowledge. However, in moving on to qualified status, the onus is on the individual to sustain their communication skills and to practise ethically. This book has emphasised the value of reflection for practitioners and here we assert that deeper theoretical appreciation enhances the ability to reflect on and analyse practice and to point the way ahead. Communication theory, particularly in relation to ethical practice, allows for an exploration of knowledge, values and behaviour. As students move into professional practice, they will need to enhance and build competence in their own communicative practice and in those they will be supervising. Arguably, the major challenges for contemporary practitioners are to maintain their ethical stances under difficult conditions and to achieve a level of communicative collaboration with patients that delivers improved outcomes. This chapter will initially define and explore the purpose of communication theory. It will go on to consider selected theoretical positions, chosen for their ability to link theory to ethical practice. We accept that there are many theoretical perspectives that are helpful and any of these could have been selected. However, within the scope of the chapter choices have to be made, so we chose to focus on Habermas, Honneth and Schön due to their focus on ethics, communication and reflective practice (other resources and further reading will be highlighted at the end of the chapter).

We begin by returning to our first two students.

Student story 13.1: Return to Janet

Janet is now a third-year student nurse. She is one of the more mature students at age 38 but has remained full of enthusiasm for her career change and still considers herself to be a 'people person'. Her family has been supportive and she is feeling positive about approaching her first post as a staff nurse. She got over her fears of having to have all the answers due to being a mature student and has thoroughly enjoyed the theory and practice. She hopes to work in an acute medical ward. However, the same bad publicity about poor standards of care that existed when she began training is still in the news. Janet recognises that much of the responsibility for raising and maintaining standards is down to people like her. She is wondering about how she will keep up her own enthusiasm and influence others to practise respectfully.

Student story 13.2: Return to Jack

Jack is a third-year learning disability student nurse. He worked as a support worker in learning disabilities prior to commencing his nursing course. He enjoyed the support work but, having almost completed his nursing course, now recognises the challenges in ensuring that people with learning disabilities are treated with dignity and respect at all times. He is very aware

(Continued)

(Continued)

that there have been a number of inquiries into poor care in hospitals for people with learning disabilities and that qualified nurses have a duty to ensure this type of abuse does not happen. In addition, there is a need to advocate for people with learning disabilities to ensure they get better access to physical healthcare. Ethical practice is a very real issue in this field of care and Jack recognises that, as a qualified nurse, he will have a responsibility to lead others and to work in collaboration with other agencies. It's much more than simply the provision of basic care.

We go on to consider some of the theoretical tools that healthcare practitioners can use to develop and reflect on practice.

Definitions

By ethical practice, we mean the ability to maintain dignity, demonstrate respect and work collaboratively with patients or service users in all situations. It involves not only medical knowledge but also moral reasoning and considerations of justice (Goethals et al., 2010).

By reflective practice, we mean the ability to reflect on action in a cyclical manner, allowing the framing and reframing of a problem to seek solutions in a systematic manner. This is influenced by Schön's (1983) account of reflection 'in action', where immediate problem solving takes place based on previous experience and knowledge, and reflection 'on action' takes place after the event (Sellars, 2014).

Theory is defined as 'temporarily accepted generalisations about the influences on and consequent variations in human action'. Theory may be constructed from philosophical positions such as that of how we determine acceptable values for behaviour or from research (Kearney, 2007, p. 148).

The importance of communication theory

In practice-based professions, it can be tempting to see theory as divorced from the reality of doing. The theory–practice gap is frequently commented on in nursing and students can get frustrated with theory. Theory may be temporary and often students are taught all about a theorist only then to be told that the theory has since been superseded by another (Silverman, 2015). Nevertheless, despite the frustrations and lack of certainty, theory, as demonstrated throughout this book, helps make sense of the world and can enable progress to be made.

CRITICAL THINKING EXERCISE 13.1
WHAT'S THE POINT OF THEORY?

Do you ever use theory in your practice?

Think of your practice placements. How have you enabled someone with a long-term condition to change health-damaging behaviour? These conditions take up 75% of the NHS budget so change is essential.

What knowledge/theories might help you to plan and support behaviour change with a patient with a long-term condition?

Remember Chapter 5 and the trans-theoretical model of change? There are theories to explain maladaptive health behaviour and how to enable positive health behaviour change.

Is it (1) effective and (2) ethical to simply leave the patient to continue to damage their health? What about diabetes and weight control?

Theories and models help with thinking and reflecting in order to make meaning of a situation. However, models are not quite the same as theories. Models represent the system being observed. They are often used in communication and certainly are used across this book to show 'how' and 'what' to communicate, but theories also explain 'why'. The world of healthcare is anything but certain and in contrast is often chaotic. Professionals need to be able to cope with uncertainty, uncover the patterns and make sense of the apparent chaos (Ghaye and Lillyman, 2014).

Hayes (2012) sees theory as a lens through which to view, leading to a map that can take things forward and change ideas into action. Hayes (2012, p. 8) argues that theory is essential to professional practice as it provides 'learnable intelligence' or the ability to see, analyse and respond to professional challenges. Without theory, rhetoric simply becomes a clashing of opinion. As student healthcare professionals approach qualification, it is helpful to consider the theoretical explanations/models that foster positive values and behaviour in communication with others. Health, healthcare and health outcomes are complex and mediated through interaction between the patient and the practitioner. As Sabater-Galindo et al. (2016) note, the relationships and interactions between practitioner and patient are the most influential factors in health outcomes, and theoretical models help explain these relationships. In order to be a compassionate and competent practitioner, it is necessary to understand one's own actions and intentionally use communicative strategies to best effect. Sabater-Galindo et al. (2016) found that theories which allowed for the exploration of patient expectations and perceptions were most useful in facilitating clear communication and better outcomes.

Rimal and Lapinski (2009, p. 247) (writing for the World Health Organization) reflect on the growing importance of communication theory in healthcare. Across the world now and not only in developed countries, behaviour that leads to obesity and associated health conditions is a major source of concern: 'Given the global challenges posed by major threats, health communication scholars and practitioners recognise the importance of prevention and, with it, the need to understand human behaviour through the prism of theory. In particular, communication theory is helpful as it is closely allied with research and with practice'. Rimal and Lapinski (2009, p. 247) argue that progress in health communication is moving in a very positive direction:

> Health communication has much to celebrate and contribute. The field is gaining recognition in part because of its emphasis on combining theory and practice in understanding communication processes and changing human behaviour. This approach is pertinent at a time when many of the threats to global public health (through diseases and environmental calamities) are rooted in human behaviour.

Therefore, communication theory is helpful on a number of levels: it enables examination as to what constitutes professional and ethical practice, it advances an understanding of communication between practitioner and patient, and helps in the modification of the health-damaging behaviour of individuals and groups.

Communication, reflective and ethical practice

Practice professions such as nursing and teaching place an emphasis on the development of reflective practice that continually examines and operates in a cycle of improvement. This can be difficult and it is tempting to neglect reflection in fast-moving and busy environments (Sellars, 2014). Reflection involves both emotional and technical aspects as technical competence is necessary for good practice but insufficient on its own. As has already been noted within this book, practitioners who do not attend to their own and others' communicative transactions and emotions run the risk of burnout (Baughan and Smith, 2013). Schön's (1983, p. 3) work, *The Reflective Practitioner*, talked about the messiness of the reality of practice in the 'swampy lowlands', where 'messy, confusing problems defy technical solutions'. This is seen in contrast to 'the high ground of research and technique', where assumptions are made that evidence-based practice will have an answer for everything. Schön asks us to acknowledge that reality and people can be difficult, potentially angry and distressed in a practice situation. There does need to be a focus on subjective feelings and on the importance of communicative transactions with one another. Schön's work on reflection chimes with recent calls for a mindful approach, criticising 'off the shelf, mindless recipes' as a method of practice (Kinsella, 2007, p. 106).

Ruedy and Schweitzer (2010) look at the use of mindfulness in ethical decision making, noting that mindfulness has the capacity to enable us to be critically observant of our own thoughts. The ability to be mindful is useful in distancing ourselves from emotion, where emotion might threaten to overwhelm. A mindful approach, centred on the present (unclouded by past memories) and focused on non-judgemental acceptance, allows decisions to be made in the light of all necessary information, rather than on the basis of placating uncomfortable emotions. Ruedy and Schweitzer's (2010) study explored the hypothesis that people who were less mindful were also less likely to make ethical decisions. They measured for mindfulness traits and concluded that those low on mindfulness also scored more lowly on moral identity and were less likely to make ethically-based decisions.

CRITICAL THINKING EXERCISE 13.2
MINDFULNESS-BASED DECISION MAKING

Think about the position of the nurses in a scandal-hit situation such as Mid Staffordshire or Winterbourne View.

At both hospitals, isolated nurses spoke up despite being bullied and urged to stay quiet by colleagues and senior staff.

Think about a situation where you faced an ethical decision. It may not have been quite so dire as those noted above, but just something where there was a dilemma between the 'right' decision and the path that the majority view seemed to favour.

What influenced your decision making?

What were your emotions and how (if you did) were you to able to make decisions despite or because of those emotions?

On analysis and reflection, what, if anything, might you have done differently and why?

Reflective and mindful practice enables ethical practice. Positive values, good communication skills and a willingness to collaborate with service users are all integral to ethical practice. As Holt and Convey (2012) noted, the NMC, when establishing codes of practice, cited professional ethics and values as a cornerstone of practice. In the updated 2015 code of ethics, the first standard states:

> You put the interests of people using or needing nursing or midwifery services first. You make their care and safety your main concern and make sure that their dignity is preserved and their needs are recognised, assessed and responded to. You make sure that those receiving care are treated with respect, that their rights are upheld and that any discriminatory attitudes and behaviours towards those receiving care are challenged. (NMC, 2015, p. 5)

It goes on say: 'Listen to people and respond to their preferences and concerns' and 'respect the level to which people receiving care want to be involved in decisions about their own health, wellbeing and care ... respect, support and document a person's right to accept or refuse care and treatment ... recognise when people are anxious or in distress and respond compassionately and politely' (NMC, 2015, p. 6).

This leaves little doubt that professional and ethical practice demands respectful behaviour and effective communication in the UK. Codes of practice in other countries also insist on similar measures (Nursing and Midwifery Board of Australia, 2008). Holt and Convey (2012) point out that ethical practice demands more than simple politeness or common courtesy. Ethical practice is concerned with moral behaviour. As discussed in Part 1, ethics and morality need to be part of the focus of communication in healthcare. Human interaction and decision making are part of nursing and involve moral reasoning. Ethical practice involves good communication, the capacity to demonstrate listening and also the ability to make competent decisions based on empathic understanding (Holt and Convey, 2012).

Communication theory that informs and enables reflection on ethical practice in healthcare

Ethical behaviour and ethical communication can sometimes be challenging. Ethical practice means according dignity and respect to patients and service users. Whereas there are many examples of professionals who exhibit respect in their dealings with patients, there are also too many accounts of poor behaviour and uncompassionate care. Martins (2005) explores how health professionals can fail to understand that the authority of their role is insufficient in achieving effective communication with patients. He discusses how advances in biotechnology have transformed certain acute and terminal illnesses, such as diabetes, into long-term and supposedly manageable conditions. Hence, the aim of healthcare practitioners has been to 'gain compliance' from the patient, making assumptions that science-based health education will persuade people to behave in appropriate ways (Martins, 2005, p. 62). However, the outcome often is that the patient does not follow instructions and is less than adherent with the prescribed medication regime. Martins notes that this approach of assuming that technical expertise and health education enable behaviour change ignores many of the conditions necessary to achieve real communication and improved outcomes. These necessary conditions include a context of mutual respect for identity.

Respect for identity

Fraser and Honneth (2003) and Honneth's (2007) theory of recognition focus on the concept of respect for identity; this is helpful in understanding the sense of injury inflicted on an individual by the persistent experience of disrespect and the process by which some come to deny respect to others. Where an individual or a number of individuals become part of a discredited group, society may devalue the identities of those within the group. A group can become discredited by their lack of relative power and this can occur in patient groups, particularly where they have long-term conditions. Charmaz (2014) has carried out much research with people with chronic or long-term conditions, highlighting how they feel they are treated as somehow being inferior. Honneth's (2007) theory explains how the process of having one's identity repeatedly deemed less worthy of respect than others becomes an experience of disrespect. Disrespect is powerful and damaging, interfering with a sense of self already acquired through socialisation and interaction with others. It is a rejection of someone's identity claim, affecting self-esteem in a very profound manner. This is similar to Goffman's classic (1961) work on the dehumanisation of psychiatric patients in the old asylums of the past. Sadly, the disappearance of the old asylums has not led to the disappearance of treating certain less powerful groups with disrespect. If people are not thought worthy of respect, they are less likely to be accorded dignity. Nordenfelt (2009, p. 35) has referred to the 'dignity of identity', no matter their class, creed, race or social position. Healthcare practice is demanding and where nurses and midwives fail to be mindful, non-judgemental and aware of their own emotional needs, they may slip into disrespectful communicative practice. If healthcare practitioners lose (or simply fail to demonstrate) respect for the identities of the people in their care, this may explain the accounts of uncompassionate care as described in relation to Mid Staffordshire Hospital and Winterbourne View. Concern about respectful and ethical practice is not limited to the UK. Brien's (2012) study concluded that ethical conflict was the most concerning element of practice for student nurses in different areas of the world.

CRITICAL THINKING EXERCISE 13.3
IDENTITY

What is your identity? How would you describe yourself?

- As you move towards qualification, think about your practice experiences.
- Think about an occasion when you nursed a patient with an identity very different from your own.
- How did you ensure the patient knew that you had respect for their identity?

Difference does not have to mean lack of respect as Patient story 13.1 from Patient Opinion demonstrates.

Patient/family story 13.1: Respect for identity

I am writing this as a family member of a person with a learning disability, to thank ****
[learning disability nurse – primary care] for all she did for my relative. My relative has several
health issues for which she needs monitoring by healthcare professionals. One aspect of that
monitoring is having regular blood tests. She is very frightened about having these taken and
becomes distressed and refuses to have them taken. **** was asked to work with her, she spent
time with her, got to know her and built up a trusting relationship. She talked her through
the tests and arranged for a phlebotomist to visit her at home. With **** and familiar support
staff around her the phlebotomist was able to successfully take the tests and she was relaxed
and not distressed. The family greatly appreciate all **** has done for her, she is an amazing,
dedicated nurse who does a wonderful job. (www.patientopinion.org.uk)

Valuing understanding as highly as technical competence

Individual identity may become less worthy of respect where professionals perceive themselves as technicians. Both Schön and Habermas write about the concern that a focus on
the technical side of practice can lead to an ignoring of the importance of good communication and subjective experience. Schön (1983) writes about the problems of assuming
the dominance of technical rationality in healthcare. There are dangers in simply following
the guidelines without reflecting on what is being done and without checking how others
are responding.

Habermas (2003) identified three types of knowledge, all of which are equally valid, but
often some types are (wrongly) judged subordinate to others.

Habermas's typology of knowledge

- Technical and scientific progress, often used within and to develop structures in the modern world
- Interpretive knowledge that strives for shared comprehension and consequently is capable of
  mobilising agreed practical action
- Knowledge that aims for mutual understanding by making useful connections between technical scientific and interpretive knowledge.

Habermas is concerned that there is a tendency to see the first type of knowledge –
technical and scientific – as superior, to the detriment of knowledge that prioritises
communication and understanding. Nurses and other healthcare professionals often
report feeling conflicted by the demands of the organisation for technical efficiency and
the emotional needs of their patients (Brien, 2012). It is suggested that in the world of
work, technical competence tends to be valued more highly as this reflects the concerns of
the organisation and the system. Habermas divides the world into the system and the
lifeworld:

- The system is the world of the organisation, the company, the government.
- The lifeworld is the world that matters to the individual: their own concerns and problems, family, culture.

Attending only to the system's needs becomes a tempting proposition in the modern world as this type of behaviour often seems to be rewarded (Habermas, 2003). However, Habermas asserts that this neglect of the individual's lifeworld concerns is exactly what causes difficulty in communication and co-operation. If we use his theory to examine many areas of healthcare, where it is essential to work collaboratively with patients, we can see that it is necessary to value the third aspect of his typology of knowledge. In order to implement technical cures, it is necessary to have the consent and co-operation of the patient. This involves understanding and mutual respect. Systems and organisations (Habermas's system) are necessary in the modern world but they often do not take account of people and their concerns, worries and preoccupations (Habermas's lifeworld). When working within these systems and organisations, we are cognisant of the goals we need to meet in order to get the job done. However, meeting the organisation's goals might not always be compatible with a patient's concerns.

Achieving mutual understanding is more difficult than it first seems

It is important to acknowledge that understanding one another is not a simple task. Habermas's Theory of Communicative Action (TCA) combines individual experience with analysis of the effects of societal power (2003). Again, it can be tempting to blame individual healthcare practitioners for disrespectful practice but the role of the external world must also be considered. Habermas is interested in how individuals and groups can reach the stage where they collaborate and treat each other with mutual respect. He argues that the structures of the world, such as organisational, economic and technological pressures, influence us to try to achieve a goal without bothering to reach agreement with the other person first (Cooke, 2002, p. 2). If collaborative decision making and reciprocal respect are to be achieved in healthcare settings, then professionals and service users must aim for a position of mutual understanding and be able to work together without power differentials and a lack of respect getting in the way.

In the modern world of healthcare that is increasingly busy and demanding, a professional has to balance an individual patient's need with that of the system. This is not an easy thing to do but awareness and understanding of the seemingly contradictory nature of the task allow the nurse to mindfully and analytically address the situation. Habermas stresses that if we wish to achieve mutual understanding, each communicative encounter must begin with that aim. This contrasts with a situation where a health professional enters the communicative encounter with the aim of achieving a specific outcome. That outcome may well be a desired state (such as healthier eating patterns) but TCA suggests that it is less likely to be reached if the professional omits the stage of reaching mutual understanding. Unless the professional actually wants to understand how the patient feels and sees their situation, any attempt at health promotion is likely to fail. Conversely, where patients recognise that the professional is really interested, they are more likely to be able to co-operate with and influence their treatment pathway (Gault et al., 2013).

Ghaye and Lillyman (2014) stress that reflective practice is the method by which we avoid falling into the technical rationality trap and lose the ability to communicate effectively with each other and critically reflect on our practice. They point out that there are many reflective models from which to choose, but they suggest that effective models contain certain types of questions.

CRITICAL THINKING EXERCISE 13.4
REFLECTION

Ask the following questions of yourself:

- Am I satisfied with how I relate to my patients? Do I want to change this? And if so, how and why?
- Does my practice reflect my values?
- Does the organisation influence me to communicate less well than I would like?
- Are my communication and practice collaborative?

CRITICAL THINKING EXERCISE 13.5
CONFLICTING PRIORITIES

Can you think of situations where the major concern of the patients seemed to be at odds with the views of the professionals?

Think of an example from practice where you felt torn between the needs of your patients and the goals of your workplace:

- How did you feel?
- What did you do?
- How did (or could) a mindful approach help to reconcile the differences?
- What factors will influence your communication in this instance? How do you reach 'mutual understanding' with your patient in this situation?

In Schön's (1983) 'swampy lowlands' of practice, thinking about, reflecting on and being mindful of the situation are crucial. Healthcare practice is challenging and stressful but also very rewarding when professionals can manage their own emotional responses and enjoy their interactions with patients. A mindful and reflective approach, aided by theoretical understanding, enhances the ability to analyse our own practice and reflexively respond and attend to patients' emotional and communicative needs. The message of Chapter 2 still stands – find a method of reflection that works for you.

Critical debate 13.1

How do you define 'ethical practice'?

Conclusion

This final chapter explored a few of the many available theoretical perspectives on communication theory and what these might offer to communication practice in healthcare. Although this might feel removed from your current practice as a student, it will become part of your role as a professional. The Australian Health Professions Council stresses that a

> **profession** is a disciplined group of individuals who adhere to ethical standards. This group positions itself as possessing special knowledge and skills in a widely recognised body of learning derived from research, education and training at a high level, and is recognised by the public as such. A profession is also prepared to apply this knowledge and exercise these skills in the interest of others. (Professions Australia – www.professions.com.au/about-us/what-is-a-professional)

This chapter focused on equipping a nurse, as they enter qualified status, with theoretical and ethical positions that invite reflection on interaction with others. The roles of theory, ethical and collaborative practice were defined and explored. It was asserted that health communication needs to be both ethical and collaborative if it is to achieve positive outcomes. Honneth's theory of respect for identity allowed us to understand the injury that persistently feeling disrespected can inflict on certain groups of patients. Habermas's (1987) theory of communicative action and Schön's of reflective practice explained how the modern world's preoccupation with technical efficiency can exert a subtle influence, leading health professionals to focus less on communication and the emotional needs of their patients. Habermas also outlined how the assumed dominance of the system downgrades individual lifeworld concerns. Consequently, professionals may not commence from a position where they wish to fully understand the patient. As a result, their health education communication may fail as mutual understanding is never achieved.

Schön's theories have been taken up by education and nursing to enable deeper and more personal reflection in action. Healthcare practice requires not only much technical efficiency but also a high level of competence in communicating with others who may be distressed and/or anxious. This book began by considering how practitioners who enter nursing and midwifery wanting to help people could reach a stage where they ignored the emotional and physical needs of their patients. We have examined ways in which nurses and midwives can increase self-awareness and emotional intelligence and learn how to look after themselves in mindful ways. However, as qualified practitioners they will also need to develop practice and lead others. This requires a deeper reflection that incorporates theoretical understanding, ethics and mindful, communicative practice.

Further suggested activity

Explore ethics in more detail – see the *Nursing Ethics* journal at http://nej.sagepub.com/
Revisit reflection with Ghaye and Lillyman (2014).
Revisit the Patients Association at www.patients-association.org.uk/ to look at how respect (or lack of it) feels for patients and service users.
Also explore the following:
Communication Theory journal – http://onlinelibrary.wiley.com/journal/10.1111/(ISSN)1468-2885
Health Communication journal – www.tandfonline.com/loi/hhth20#.VxK00TArLIU

Health Expectations journal – http://onlinelibrary.wiley.com/journal/10.1111/(ISSN)1369-7625
Professions Australia, 'What is a profession?' – www.professions.com.au/about-us/what-is-a-professional

To access further resources related to this chapter, visit the Values Exchange website at http://
sagecomms.vxcommunity.com

References

Baughan, J. and Smith, A. (2013) *Compassion, Caring and Communication*, 2nd edn. London: Pearson Education.

Brien, S. (2012) 'Beyond Competence' literature review: final report. University of Southampton, 31 October. Available at: www.southampton.ac.uk/assets/imported/transforms/content-block/UsefulDownloads_Download/6097118CD76042B1926932B0FD7106D2/BC%20Literature%20review%20Soton%20Nursing.pdf (accessed 16 April 2016).

Charmaz, C. (2014) *Constructing Grounded Theory*. Thousand Oaks, CA: Sage.

Cooke, M. (ed.) (2002) *On the Pragmatics of Communication*. Cambridge: Polity.

Fraser, N. and Honneth, A. (2003) *Redistribution or Recognition: A Political-Philosophical Exchange*. London: Verso.

Gault, I., Gallagher, A. and Chambers, M. (2013) 'Perspectives on medicine adherence in service users and carers with experience of legally sanctioned detention and medication: a qualitative study', *Patient Preference and Adherence*, 7: 787–99.

Ghaye, T. and Lillyman, S. (2014) *Reflection: Principles and Practices for Healthcare Professionals*, 2nd edn. London: Quay Books/Mark Allen Group.

Goethals, S., Gastmans, C. and Dierckx de Casterle, B. (2010) 'Nurses' ethical reasoning and behaviour: a literature review', *International Journal of Nursing Studies*, 45: 635–50.

Goffman, E. (1961) *Asylums*. New York: Anchor Books.

Habermas, J. (1987) *The Theory of Communicative Action*, Vol. 2. Boston, MA: Beacon Press.

Habermas, J. (2003) *On the Pragmatics of Communication*. Cambridge: Polity Press.

Hayes, V. (2012) 'From Page to Practice: Communication Theory and its Value for Public Relations Educators and Practitioners'. Unpublished MA thesis, Royal Roads University, Toronto (accessible at www.researchgate.net/).

Holt, J. and Convey, H. (2012) 'Ethical practice in nursing care', *Nursing Standard*, 27(13): 51–6.

Honneth, A. (2007) *Disrespect: The Normative Foundations of Critical Theory*, 2nd edn. Cambridge: Polity Press.

Kearney, M. (2007) 'From the sublime to the meticulous: the continuing evolution of grounded formal theory', in A. Bryant and K. Charmaz (eds), *The Sage Handbook of Grounded Theory*. London: Sage. pp. 127–50.

Kinsella, E. (2007) 'Technical rationality in Schön's reflective practice: dichotomous or non-dualistic epistemological position', *Nursing Philosophy*, 8(2): 102–13.

Martins, D. (2005) 'Compliance rhetoric and the impoverishment of context', *Communication Theory*, 15(1): 59–77.

Nordenfelt, L. (2004) 'The varieties of dignity', *Health Care Analysis*, 12(2): 69–89.

Nordenfelt, L. (ed.) (2009) *Dignity in Care for Older People*. Oxford: Wiley Blackwell.

Nursing and Midwifery Council (NMC) (2015) *Code of Ethics*. London: NMC.

Nursing and Midwifery Board of Australia (2008) *Code of Professional Conduct for Nurses in Australia*. Melbourne: Nursing and Midwifery Board of Australia.

Rimal, R. and Lapinski, M. (2009) 'Why health communication is important in public health', *Bulletin of the World Health Organization*, 87: 247.

Ruedy, N.E. and Schweitzer, M.E. (2010) 'In the Moment: The Effect of Mindfulness on Ethical Decision Making', Russell Ackoff Fellowship of the Wharton Risk Center, University of

Pennsylvania, Working Paper No. 2010-07-02, July. Available at: http://opim.wharton.upenn.edu/risk/library/WPAF2010-07-02_NR,MS.pdf (accessed 16 April 2016).

Sabater-Galindo, M., Fernandoz-Limos, F., Sabater-Martinez, D., Martinez-Martinez, F. and Benrimoj, S. (2016) 'Healthcare professional–patient relationships: systematic review of theoretical models from a community pharmacy perspective', *Patient Education and Counseling*, 99(3): 339–47.

Schön, D. (1983) *The Reflective Practitioner.* New York: Basic Books.

Sellars, M. (2014) *Reflective Practice for Teachers.* London: Sage.

Silverman, D. (2015) *Doing Qualitative Research: A Practical Handbook*, 4th edn. London: Sage.

CONCLUSION
TO
PART 3

Part 3 has considered some of the more difficult and thorny problems that confront health professionals working in pressured environments. The priorities of organisations and the necessity to manage the shift may, at times, seem to clash with giving enough emotional attention to patients. When confronted with this reality, some practitioners have been unable to maintain and sustain compassionate communication with their patients. However, many others do and it is this that we have examined in order to consider what it is that helps professionals maintain the caring attitudes with which they entered the profession. Organisations should not be let off the hook and enlightened management can recognise and respond to their role in looking after staff (however, that is another book for another time).

Looking after oneself is crucial when dealing with the intense emotional demands of healthcare. This is not weakness but a practical and sensible approach to maintaining optimum functioning in stressful circumstances. There is no single prescription for the type of supervision or support that works most effectively but there are a number of models that have proved successful. Healthcare organisations have a duty to provide preceptorship and support, so constructively and assertively requesting such supervision will be helpful for all.

Understanding the nature of organisations, how the prevailing culture can affect the team's performance and the ability to support one another, is crucial if that culture needs to change and/or improve. Understanding our own responses and developing the ability to manage our responses is also essential to prevent moral disengagement or burnout.

Lastly, after the initial transition period, you will be part of a profession that has the ability and responsibility to think through and develop ethical and communicative practice. We do not insist that the theories examined within this book are the only or the most appropriate theories to help take communicative and collaborative practice forward, but we do suggest they are a good start.

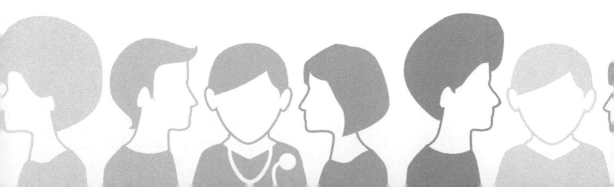

Index

emotional competence 45
emotional intelligence (EI) 44–6, 138
emotional labour (EL) 148–9, 150
emotional mind 42, 46
emotional wellbeing
　of nurses and midwives 13
empathic curiosity 88
empathic listening 88
empathy 7, 68
　definition 88
Encyclopaedia Britannica 102
end-of-life care 120
end-of-life conditions 119–22
　palliative care 120
　softly softly approach 120
epinephrine 33
equilibrium 28
ethical decision making 160
ethical practice 158, 161
expressive caring 138
expressive language/communication 84

facilitative interventions 77
familiarity 83
family-centred care (FCC) 92
　definition 92
　triad of communication 93
family, the
　communicating within the context of
　　92–5
feeling rules 150
feelings 23
five As of anger deflection 114–15
fluid intelligence 105
formal operational stage 29
Francis Report 6, 106, 131, 152
Fraser, N. and Honneth, A. 9, 162
frontal brain 31
funding 6

GABA (gamma aminobutryc acid) 33
Gabe, J. 150
Gallagher, A. 9
Garwood-Gowers et al. 10
gerotranscendence 109
Gerson et al. 34
Ghaye, T. 22, 23
Ghaye, T. and Lillyman, S. 23, 165
Gibbs's reflective cycle 23
Gillick competence 97
Goffman, Erving 69
Goleman, Daniel 44, 45
Goodman, B. 149, 150, 152
Goodrich, J. 153
Groves et al. 60

Habermas, Jürgen 163–4, 166
Happell, B. 10

Hayes, V. 159
health behaviour
　change 41–4, 60–6
　long-term conditions (LTCs) 61
　positive 38–48, 62
Health Care Leadership Model 135
health education 39–40
　definition 39
healthcare education
　collaborative decision making 41
　information 41
healthcare professionals
　communication behaviour 7–8
　communication styles 95
　public confidence in 21
Heron, John 77
Hibbard, J.H. and Greene, J. 40
hierarchical, organisational culture 132
hippocampus 32
Hochschild, A.R. 150
Hollinrake, S. 150
Holt, J. and Convey, H. 161
Honneth, A. 162, 166
hope 120–1
Huang et al. 34
hypothalamus 31, 32

iatrogenic care 108
identity 9
　professional 21–2
　respect for 162, 166
Ikeda et al. 34
ill health, changing patterns of 39–40
illness
　psychosocial care and 56
　stress of 113
indignity 8
individual discrimination 71
infants
　crying 96
　developing communication skills 96
institutionalisation 108
instrumental caring 138
intellectual disability
　ability to communicate 81
　Augmentative and Alternative Communication
　　(AAC) strategies 84–5
　communication needs 82–4
　definition 82
　stigma 82
intelligence 105
Intensive Interaction 85
Internet 98

Jack et al. 59, 60
jargon 17
Johnson et al. 21
Jung, Carl 101

Hollinrake, S. (2013) 'Informal Care' in Monaghan, L. and Gabe J. (eds), *Key Concepts in Medical Sociology*. London: Sage.

Kramer, M. (1974) *Reality Shock: Why Nurses Leave Nursing*. St Louis, MO: Mosby.

Msiska, G., Smith, P. and Fawcett, T. (2014) 'Exposing emotional labour experienced by nursing students during their clinical learning experience: a Malawian perspective', *International Journal of Africa Nursing Sciences*, 1: 43–50.

Sawbridge, Y. and Hewison, A. (2011) 'Time to care? Responding to concerns about poor nursing care'. HSMC Policy Paper 12, Health Services Management Centre, University of Birmingham. Available at: www.birmingham.ac.uk/Documents/college-social-sciences/social-policy/HSMC/publications/PolicyPapers/policy-paper-twelve-time-to-care.pdf

Smith, P. (2012) *The Emotional Labour of Nursing Re-visited* (2nd edn). Hampshire: Palgrave Macmillan.

Townsend, T. (2012) 'Break the bullying cycle: we can do it through individual accountability, a mentoring culture, and support for nursing peers', *American Nurse Today*, 7(1). Available at: https://americannursetoday.com/break-the-bullying-cycle/ (accessed 16 April 2016).

Wallbank, S. and Preece, E. (2010) *Evaluation of Clinical Supervision given to Health Visitor and School Nurse Leadership Participants*. Birmingham: NHS West Midlands and Worcester University.

Whitehead, B. (2011) 'Are newly qualified nurses prepared for practice?', *Nursing Times*, 11(107): 19–20.

Zimbardo, P. G. (2004) 'A situationist perspective on the psychology of evil: understanding how good people are transformed into perpetrators', in G. Millar (ed.), *The Social Psychology of Good and Evil*. New York: Guildford Press, pp. 21–50.

Useful websites

Care Quality Commission home page: Supporting Information and Guidance: Supporting Effective Clinical Supervision – www.cqc.org.uk/

www.nhsemployers.org/your.../preceptorships-for-newly-qualified-staff www.evidence.nhs.uk/Search?q=clinical+supervision+for+nurses

To access further resources related to this chapter, visit the Values Exchange website at http:// sagecomms.vxcommunity.com